"In the third text using his Master Conflict Theory, Dr. Betchen illustrates how to deal with unmet sexual and relational expectations in conflicted couples. Betchen is masterful in integrating psychodynamic and systemic protocols, producing another valuable resource for beginning and expert clinicians alike."

Nancy Gambescia, *PhD, Former Director, Post-Graduate Sex Therapy Program, Council for Relationships, Philadelphia, Pennsylvania*

"In *Unmet Expectations*, Dr. Betchen masterfully synthesizes theory and practice into a highly important text addressing the core issues of what brings couples into treatment. Replete with diverse clinical examples, he outlines a well-constructed, comprehensive process by which therapists most effectively can conceptualize and implement Master Conflict Theory step-by-step. This is a must-have for a therapist at any stage of practice."

Katherine Hertlein, *PhD, Department of Psychiatry and Behavioral Health, University of Nevada, Las Vegas*

"In *Unmet Expectations*, Betchen uses his Master Conflict Theory to explain why some couples continue to fall short of what they want and how they pull unsuspecting therapists into the same unsatisfying pursuit. In his usual insightful way, Betchen cuts through the confusion to explain the dynamics at work for both romantic partners and how a therapist can skillfully offer these clients the ability to grow beyond the limits of their past. And, as with the rest of his writing, it is rich with clinical acumen that will make you a better therapist with both couples and individuals."

Ari Tuckman, PsyD, *author* ADHD After Dark: Better Sex Life, Better Relationship

Unmet Expectations in Couple and Sex Therapy

Stephen J. Betchen illuminates unmet expectations as one of the leading causes of relationship problems, offering an integrative, systemic, and conflict-oriented treatment model that will help both therapists and couples develop happier and more realistic relationships.

This clinical guide helps therapists provide couples with the ability to recognize the origin of their expectations and when their expectations might be realistically or unrealistically too high or low. It defines and demonstrates the complexity of what met or unmet expectations are, identifying common symptoms as anger, incessant bickering, anxiety, disappointment, disillusionment, and sadness. Chapters outline how to determine the origin and impact of unmet expectations before discussing how and why we choose our partners that do or do not meet our needs. Addressing sociocultural factors in depth, Betchen provides tools to assess and treat both sexual and non-sexual symptoms and includes a chapter on how to manage the issue of when a therapist doesn't meet the expectations of their clients.

The book is invaluable for therapists who work with couples as well as trainees and supervisors in couple, family, and sex therapy graduate and post-graduate programs.

Stephen J. Betchen, DSW, LMFT, is an AAMFT-approved supervisor and AASECT certified supervisor. He currently maintains a full-time private practice in New Jersey specializing in couples and sex therapy.

Unmet Expectations in Couple and Sex Therapy

Helping Couples Negotiate Realistic Relationships

Stephen J. Betchen

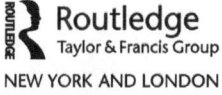
Routledge
Taylor & Francis Group

NEW YORK AND LONDON

Designed cover image: © Getty Images

First published 2024
by Routledge
605 Third Avenue, New York, NY 10158

and by Routledge
4 Park Square, Milton Park, Abingdon, Oxon, OX14 4RN

Routledge is an imprint of the Taylor & Francis Group, an informa business

Library of Congress Cataloging-in-Publication Data
Names: Betchen, Stephen J., 1954– author.
Title: Unmet expectations in couple and sex therapy: helping couples
negotiate realistic relationships / Stephen J. Betchen.
Description: New York, NY : Routledge, 2024. |
Includes bibliographical references and index.
Identifiers: LCCN 2023018148 (print) | LCCN 2023018149 (ebook) |
ISBN 9781032417301 (hardback) | ISBN 9781032417295 (paperback) |
ISBN 9781003359470 (ebook)
Subjects: LCSH: Sex therapy. | Couples therapy. | Marital psychotherapy.
Classification: LCC RC557 .B48 2024 (print) |
LCC RC557 (ebook) | DDC 616.89/1562–dc23/eng/20230607
LC record available at https://lccn.loc.gov/2023018148
LC ebook record available at https://lccn.loc.gov/2023018149

ISBN: 978-1-032-41730-1 (hbk)
ISBN: 978-1-032-41729-5 (pbk)
ISBN: 978-1-003-35947-0 (ebk)

DOI: 10.4324/9781003359470

Typeset in Times New Roman
by Newgen Publishing UK

Helen Singer Kaplan, Elisabeth Young-Bruehl and
Najla Kowalewski

*— Three esteemed women whose personal words of encouragement
gave me the confidence to both practice and write.*

Contents

About the Author

Stephen J. Betchen, DSW, is a licensed marriage and family therapist and a certified sex therapist. He completed his doctorate at the University of Pennsylvania with a specialization in marriage and family therapy and trained at Penn's Marriage Council of Philadelphia. He followed with a post-doctoral fellowship at the New York Hospital-Cornell University Medical Center's Payne Whitney Clinic in psychology (sex therapy), a clinical psychoanalytic fellowship (classical) at the Institute of the Philadelphia Association for Psychoanalysis, and study at the William Alanson White Institute in their Intensive Psychoanalytic Psychotherapy Program. Dr. Betchen is the author of several scholarly articles and chapters, magazine pieces and blogs, over 500 newspaper columns, and six books on relationships. He is an AAMFT-approved supervisor and an AASECT diplomate and certified supervisor and a former adjunct clinical professor in the Department of Couple and Family Therapy at Thomas Jefferson University and senior supervisor in the post-graduate Sex Therapy Program at the Council for Relationships. He currently writes a monthly blog on relationships for *PsychologyToday.com* and maintains a full-time private practice specializing in couples/sex therapy in Cherry Hill, New Jersey.

Acknowledgments

My thanks to those couples who have shared their expectations, met and unmet, with me over the years. Without them this book would never have been written. I would also like to thank Heather Evans at Routledge who has now served as editor for my third consecutive book. I could not have asked for anyone more supportive and open to innovative ideas.

Preface

This is the third book on Master Conflict Theory (MCT) published by Routledge, although each stand on its own. The first book, *Master Conflict Therapy: A New Model for Practicing Couples and Sex Therapy* (co-authored), outlines the foundation of the model, which was specifically designed to treat couples, and its origins in Pre-Socratic Western Philosophy and the Greek theory of opposites. The second book, *Couples in Conflict: Clinical Techniques for Navigating Sexual and Relationship Control Struggles*, applies MCT to chronic control struggles in couples. This third book, *Unmet Expectations in Couple and Sex Therapy: Helping Couples Negotiate Realistic Relationships*, demonstrates the use of the MCT model in working with couples who are conflicted about what to expect from their relationships.

After writing the foundation book, I was mainly interested in exploring those issues that are common to couples but have received only scant attention in the couples therapy literature. Almost every book on couples therapy mentions the concepts of "control" and "expectations," but no therapist or theoretician that I am aware of has dedicated an entire book to either subject.

By examining control and expectations from the perspective of conflict, these concepts can be seen in all their complexity, yet are much more understandable and treatable. When applying conflict theory, it suddenly makes sense why someone who claims to want control might also give it up or reject it, and why an individual with certain expectations might also block them from being fulfilled. These individuals are in conflict about their desires. A part of them needs these desires fulfilled and part of them is uncomfortable achieving this. The counterintuitive conflict theory approach explains, better than any other theory, why couples are stuck with symptoms for years. As a colleague once said about the model: "It makes sense of the nonsense."

Because I have always believed that every couples therapist should have sex therapy training and *vice versa*, MCT is designed to treat those couples with sexual and nonsexual problems. It has never made sense to me that marriage and family therapy are inextricably linked whereas couples and sex therapy are not. Families rarely report for therapy because of sexual problems, but this is a common occurrence for couples.

The master conflict approach is an integrative, systemic approach. And I believe that it is the most inclusive model available to treat couples. It can be applied equally to couples regardless of age, race, ethnicity, sexual orientation/ identity, and to a wide array of problems. In this book, I deal exclusively with both therapist and couples' expectations in a sexual and nonsexual context. The following material is included in this compact but comprehensive text:

- Section I: Understanding the Expectations of Couples – in "Chapter 1. Introduction: Complexity and Conflict," I define the concept of "expectation" in the context of relationships and address the consequences that can occur when they go unmet. Because expectations exist on a continuum, I address several types of expectations (e.g., Realistic Expectations-High; Unrealistic Expectations-Low). And finally, I examine expectations from a conflict theory perspective.
- "Chapter 2. The Origin of Expectations," explores how expectations are generated. This chapter covers the early research on the mother-infant bond espoused in the psychoanalytic literature of Sigmund and Anna Freud, Melanie Klein, Donald Winnicott, and John Bowlby, as well as in the systemic family of origin work of Murray Bowen. The chapter ends with the MCT model, which has already been established in the literature by the author.
- In "Chapter 3. Mate Choice and Expectations," I explain how partners choose each other based on a shared conflict around expectations.
- In "Chapter 4. Sociocultural Influences," I demonstrate the pervasiveness of the concept of expectations by its application to couples of various cultures (e.g., American-Born Man and American-Born Greek Woman; Israeli-Born Man and Israeli-Born Woman). Race, religion, and sexual orientation are also considered in the context of conflicts and expectations.
- Section II: Clinical Assessment of Expectations – "Chapter 5. Assessing Couples with Unmet Expectations." helps the couples therapist assess the symptoms of unmet expectations, nonsexual and sexual. The Genogram is the assessment tool used in this process. I include sample questions specifically aimed at helping the therapist assess a couple's conflict with expectations and use two detailed cases to illustrate the assessment process.
- Section III: Clinical Treatment – "Chapter 6. Treating Couples with Unmet Expectations," demonstrates the use of the MCT model to treat couples suffering from symptoms, nonsexual and sexual, because of an unbalanced conflict around expectations. The model is made up of a 5-step treatment process which includes the uncovering of the couple's shared conflict and the differentiation process used to balance or rebalance it. Sexual exercises and case examples are included.

• "Chapter 7. The Therapist's Expectations," explores the therapist's own conflicts around expectations, suggesting that to maximize the effectiveness of the MCT approach, it would be helpful for the couples therapist to have experienced personal psychotherapy. Without this background, the therapist is more likely to have an unbalanced conflict around expectations that may exacerbate or further unbalance the conflicts of those couples in treatment.

Section I

Understanding the Expectations of Couples

1   Introduction

Complexity and Conflict

Consequences

The word expectation comes from the Latin word *expectationem*, meaning "an awaiting." It is defined as a belief about what might happen in the future. It can also denote something that is supposed to happen (Harris, 2008). Given my work as a couples therapist, it was not long before I became curious about expectations in the context of couples. And in doing so, I discovered that it proved to be a major cause of meaningful relationship problems. Several studies have substantiated my findings (Bian, 2021; Kabra, 2019; Kloppers, 2021), including a large-scale survey of approximately 1,500 Americans conducted between 2003 and 2004 by the National Fatherhood Initiative (2005). The results of the survey indicated that approximately 45% of husband-and-wife respondents attributed unrealistic expectations to the cause of their divorce.

In my clinical work I have heard countless partners express a host of potentially destructive feelings associated with unmet expectations in their relationships such as: anger, anxiety, disappointment, and depression. These reactions are most often related to money (e.g., "You don't work hard enough or make enough money"); family participation (e.g., "You don't spend enough time with the family"); a lack of affection (e.g., "You never hold my hand or kiss me hello. I do not think you are attracted to me anymore"); and a significant discrepancy in sexual frequency (e.g., "We never have enough sex. And you never initiate it"); sexual quality (e.g., "There is no foreplay, you go right to intercourse"); and sexual openness (e.g., "You never want to experiment with anything new. It is always the same old boring missionary style sex").

When accompanied by anger, unmet expectations are usually representative of partners who perceive that their counterparts are purposely refusing to meet their needs. Rarely do I hear "You cannot satisfy me." Instead, I hear "You won't satisfy me," or "You refuse to give me what I want." Many of these complaints are merited, in part, because it is easy for couples to be consciously or unconsciously locked into a cycle of mutual retaliation. But there can be a legitimate reason one partner cannot satisfy the other and too often the disappointed partner rarely considers this as a "good enough" excuse. For example, Ellen's husband Bill suffered a stroke and he claimed that he could no longer work. Ellen saw his stroke as mild and so after a few months of rehabilitation she began to pester him

DOI: 10.4324/9781003359470-2

to get a job. After years of her haranguing and his passive aggressive behavior, a psychiatrist Bill consulted diagnosed him with severe depression. To the chagrin of his wife, the psychiatrist told her that given his condition Bill was not able to hold a job.

Unmet expectations can cause anxiety. This is especially true for those people who enter a relationship with expectations of security and stability. If they happen to find that their partner has a problem that threatens their security, anxiety will follow. For example, a young woman whose father lost all the family money because of his poor business decisions began to experience panic attacks when she discovered that her husband had a gambling problem. She quickly filed for divorce.

A male client, Kurt, reported to treatment disillusioned. He said that Risa, his girlfriend – who he was planning to marry – suddenly broke up with him because he had lost his job. He told her that he had been looking for new employment, but she did not believe him. Claiming he was blindsided, Kurt implored Risa to better explain her concerns. In a painful and embarrassing moment, Risa admitted that her father was a terrible provider; a "lazy man" who saw little value in financial security. As a result, Risa's family was left to cope with an ever-present anxiety which impacted her deeply. Risa promised herself that she would never relive the experience if, and when, she married. Risa also added that Kurt was not looking hard enough for work and seemed "too content" with his current state of unemployment. Kurt expected a bit more empathy from Risa. In contrast, Risa expected Kurt to be frantic about losing his job and to do everything in his power to get another one as soon as possible.

Unmet expectations may cause disappointment and depression – one partner feels let down by the other. But ironically, the partner who fails the other may feel disappointment in him or herself… even tremendous guilt. A male client who experienced a demanding, yet emotionally neglectful set of parents long exhibited a harsh superego. As an older adult he developed erectile disorder (ED) and felt so guilty and disappointed in his inability to perform that he gave his young wife permission to find a young man to service her – at least until he gained control of his problem.

Expectations that go unmet can also "shock" a partner, upending the individual's "sense of world order." For example, a young wife was extremely upset by her husband's affair. A religious woman, she could not believe he would do such a thing, even though he admitted it. She became obsessed with trying to figure out what the truth was while simultaneously rejecting it.

Despite unfulfilled expectations, even of the most traumatic kind, some couples remain loyal to each other. These individuals claim to be looking for some slight change or a mild adjustment in their counterpart's behavior which they consider "doable." In some cases, it can be that simple, but in most this way of thinking turns out to be a fantasy that only helps to maintain the couple's dynamic. It is also one of the main reasons we see partners traumatized by the same unmet expectation repeatedly, even if they are pre-warned.

A middle-aged husband proved to be a serial cheater. In approximately fifteen years of marriage, he had fourteen known affairs. And every time he was caught with a new lover his wife would claim to be devastated. Even though she knew of his record, experienced the pain of his transgressions repeatedly, and was warned to be careful by many, she acted as if each new affair was the first. She needed to expect a different outcome. Like this woman, some individuals believe that if only their partner would try a little harder to please them, life would vastly improve. Others believe they have chosen the wrong partner and demand they change to save the relationship. Still others question whether their chosen partner is even capable of satisfying them. "Should I have chosen someone richer, smarter, more attractive, or better in bed? Should I have found someone who is easier to please, rather than someone who always is moving the goal posts?"

Pervasiveness

Aside from its potential to cause severe problems in a relationship, I also found unmet expectations to be a pervasive concept in two distinct ways. First, I found it to exist in all couples regardless of age, race, gender identity, and sexual orientation. And while the expectations might be different in context, people still react depending on where they are on a continuum. For example, a twenty-eight-year-old newly married woman planned to start a family before she turned thirty. Her husband initially agreed to these terms but soon after marriage changed his mind. He wanted to wait for his business to become more stable, which would have conservatively taken another three to four years. Predictably the couple's disparity created tension in the relationship. The wife expected her husband to keep his word and to try and have children within two years of marriage, and the husband expected his wife to be more flexible and understanding.

By contrast an older married female client, Ruth, was not concerned with having children because hers were grown and married. She did, however, feel a strong need to live near them and her grandchildren. She expected her husband, Donald, to feel the same, but he wanted to buy a trailer so that they could tour the country. Donald said: "All Ruth ever said was that she could not wait for the kids to grow up so we could travel more freely. She is aware of how hard I worked to reach retirement. She knows how important this is to me." Ruth said that she understood her husband's position. But having grandchildren changed everything for her, and she expected him to feel the same way.

Another example includes a lesbian couple in their early forties. Jane, a mother of two boys from her marriage to a straight man, thought that her new partner Allison would value being a parent. Allison implied as much, but after a few months of living together Allison decided to end the relationship. Her reason was that she did not expect raising children to be so hard. She also admitted that she expected Jane to carry the load. Jane expected Allison to make a lifetime commitment and to share equally in raising the children.

A second reason expectations may be pervasive is because they tend to exist in different contexts. Those that expect too much from a spouse also might expect too much from employees and friends. The level of intensity might differ depending on the significance of the context, but this usually depends on where these individuals fall on the expectation continuum. For example, a woman who demanded that her husband cater to her every whim expected her friends to respond to her needs in kind. While she often scolded her husband when he disappointed her, she punished others passive-aggressively – she would shun them for long periods of time. While two distinctive styles of reacting to unmet expectations, they are similar in their levels of intensity.

Despite the pervasiveness of expectations and the enormous challenge they present to clinicians who work with couples, the concept has received scant attention in the popular literature (Beall, 2016; Chapman, 2015; DiDonato, 2017; Gottman & Silver, 2015; Grace, 2015; Harris, 2008; Hendrix & Hunt, 2019; Newbold, 2020; Perel, 2017), and even less so in the professional literature (Baker et al., 2017; Blair & Madigan, 2016; Casale et al., 2019; Khazan, 2017; Vunnier & O'Sullivan, 2018). In fact, I have not found one professional book written exclusively on the topic even though most systemic books tend to touch on the issue (Betchen, 2010, 2022; Betchen & Davidson, 2018; Betchen & Gambescia, 2020; Gambescia et al., 2021; Hertlein et al., 2020; Johnson, 2019; Nelson, 2020).

The importance of expectations in the lives of couples and the limited attention given to clinicians are the main reasons for authoring this book. Specifically, couples need to better understand the role that this concept plays in their relationships and any associated symptoms, and to learn to expect what is appropriate and realistic. Clinicians need to develop specific functional strategies to help them do so.

Complexity

The Continuum

As mentioned, because expectations vary, they are viewed on a continuum. Those at one end are people who have low expectations. This might include individuals who have little faith in life's potential for reciprocity. These people may possess feelings of resignation as if to say: "What is the point?" But this end of the continuum might also include the undeserving, or those who, real or imagined, see themselves as victims or martyrs. For example, a woman whose husband was admittedly having an affair could not seem to do anything about it. Rather than change her situation she seemed to prefer obsessively lamenting about her plight. When I questioned whether she saw a way out, she said only her husband could help. He needed to give up his lover and all would be fine again; something he was not interested in doing.

At the other end of the continuum are those with high expectations or those who expect too much given the situation and context. These individuals tend to feel they deserve to get their needs met while others may feel entitled (Boszormenyi-Nagy & Spark, 1973) to have them met. For example, a male client, Art, felt that he could buy whatever he wanted regardless of the price or necessity and without consulting his wife. He also demanded sex every night from her even when she was ill and would throw a tantrum if rejected. Art was eventually fired from his job because he was constantly harassing his boss for raises and promotions. When his wife expressed concern about their finances, Art simply told her to get a second job until he found a new one.

In my clinical experience, people rarely exist at the "extreme" opposite ends of the continuum. All people have expectations whether they voice them or not – it is human nature. Even the greatest martyr has at least one fantasy. Likewise, I have yet to find an individual who expects to have their needs met all the time in every context, even though they may express dissatisfaction. Given this, "high" and "low" are at ends of the continuum for our purposes. Note in Figure 1.1 that Keith and Joyce are opposites in their expectations. Keith is the most expectant of the two and Joyce is least expectant. Still, neither partner is at the "very ends" of the continuum of expectations. Also note that Patty appears more demanding than Sam and Joyce, but less demanding than Keith.

When I first began to consider writing about expectations, I conceived the concept as dependent on the seriousness and significance of the context. For example, a spouse would expect more positive reinforcement from a partner than from a neighbor. And one would react more strongly if a close friend failed to help in a time of need, compared to a distant cousin. While this thinking still has merit, it is a more accurate measure of a couple's expectations to "first" determine where each partner was on the expectation continuum. What might be a serious breach or disappointment can be dismissed by someone who expects little. And the smallest, most insignificant experience can be exaggerated by someone who expects a great deal. Again, this is not to say that I discount the impact of context on expectations. While those closer to the extreme ends of the continuum will overreact or underreact no matter the context or importance, the majority of those that lie in the middle prove to be more context dependent. These people tend to be less reactive in general and are better able to inter-pret their experiences in the relationship and the world more rationally and realistically.

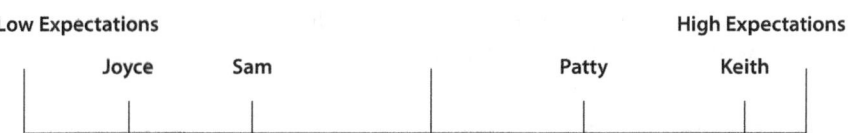

Low Expectations   **High Expectations**

    Joyce   Sam   Patty   Keith

Figure 1.1   Continuum of Expectations.

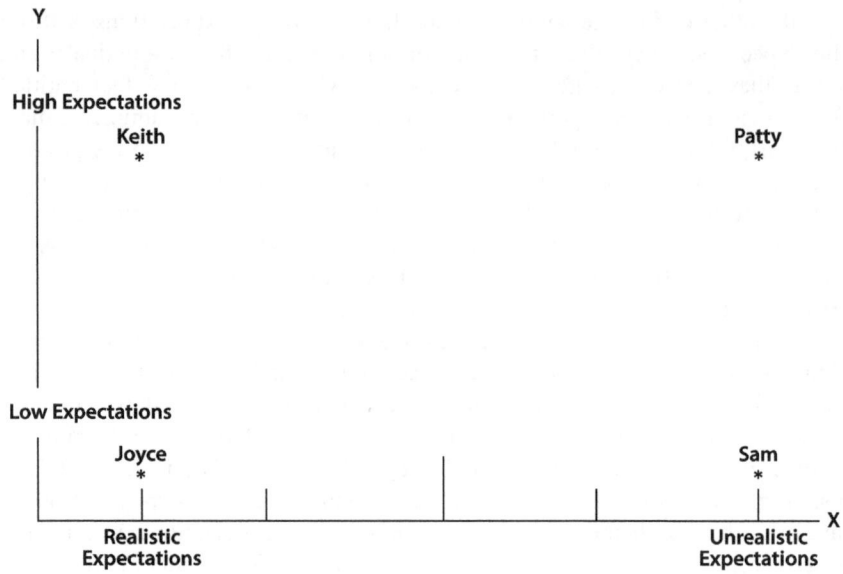

Figure 1.2   Types of Expectations.

Types

To add to the complexity, not only can those who have high expectations in relationships produce symptoms, those who have low expectations can as well. To control this, I have identified two major types of expectations: realistic and unrealistic, and examined each at both ends of the continuum. That is, when an individual has realistically high or low expectations and when an individual has unrealistically high or low expectations.

Notice in Figure 1.2 that the two major types of expectations mentioned (i.e., realistic, and unrealistic expectations) are independent variables on the x-axis while two dependent variables (i.e., high, and low expectations) are on the y-axis. Individuals can plot with realistic or unrealistic expectations on the high or low axis. Others fall in between each of the two axes and are more indicative of a balanced conflict. This is therefore less likely to cause relationship symptoms.

It is important for the clinician to use these variables to identify a couple's conflict with expectations and to accurately help balance or rebalance it. They are also helpful in understanding what compelled mate choice (see Chapter 3, Mate Choice and Expectations). Examples of all four combinations of variables that follow are in the context of relationships:

Realistic Expectations-High

People who have realistic expectations, high or low, are rational individuals who tend to have a particularly good reason to believe that their expectations will or will not be met. Some of these people may have been promised something, or even signed a contract to that end. Others know by experience that their expectations are realistic in part based on the credibility of the people they are dealing with as well as the circumstances and context. Their expectations are logical and rational. Having justifiable expectations does not guarantee that someone will or will not get their expectations met. It only suggests that the expectations are within reason. Consider the following individual with realistically high expectations:

Keith was the youngest of five siblings and the only male. His older sisters doted on him as did his parents. In growing up Keith sought out females older than he and expected to be taken care of. If they failed him, however, he would experience conflicting feelings: rage, followed by anxiety related to a fear of loss.

Keith had enough personal experience and insight to know what he needed in life. He wanted an older, competent woman who could meet his high demands. He once had a torrid love affair with an older female college professor. But he knew that he would have to play fair and try to meet her needs as well. Keith married a nurturing, local lawyer, Amanda, to whom he was pleased with and devoted to. Keith was realistic in his choice of partner.

Realistic Expectations-Low

People with low expectations also can be realistic. These people expect little in their relationships and in life in general, and many of them are justifiably realistic in their beliefs. The people in this category are in situations in which there is little hope for change or improvement and in some cases, they are reminded of this repeatedly. These individuals are completely realistic in expecting little. This does not mean that they do not deserve better. Rather, it means that the situation or context they are in is inflexible. The following case depicts an individual with realistically low expectations:

Joyce's boyfriend, Alex, warned her that he did not want children. He had two adult children from his first marriage and did not enjoy the experience. He was a self-proclaimed bad father. Alex said that he realized that he was a selfish man and wanted the option to do as he pleased with the least amount of burden. Joyce was several years younger than Alex and this was her first marriage.

Although Joyce said she would like children, she knew that Alex was immovable on this subject and acquiesced. The couple married and although the marriage was a solid one, Joyce carried with her a mild to moderate depression. When questioned about her plight she said that she knew from the beginning that Alex would never change his mind about starting a family. She admitted that she wanted more out of life but accepted less because she knew that if she wanted Alex, she had little choice in the matter. She was absolutely justified in expecting little in this context from her husband.

Unrealistic Expectations-High

People with unrealistic expectations, high or low, are gamblers. Even though the odds are against their expectations being met they wager heavily they will be. Often these individuals miss or pay little attention to verbal and behavioral cues, signs, or warnings that their expectations are closer to fantasy than reality. Some even make up their own reality; others simply fail to acknowledge a pattern that might suggest that they will never get what they are after. Unfortunately, many of these types of people often experience personal and/or professional catastrophe. Consider the following individual who had unrealistically high expectations:

Patty complained that when she and her boyfriend Terry went out on dates he would stare at other women. He even stared at her friends and her mother, all of whom reported feeling quite uncomfortable. Patty, fully conscious of Terry's behavior, was clearly disturbed by it. But she claimed that all Terry needed was to have regular sex which she planned to provide once they married. Following marriage, Patty initiated sex, but this did nothing to stop Terry from intently looking at other women. In this sense, Patty underestimated the power of Terry's pattern.

Unrealistic Expectations-Low

Some people with unrealistic expectations "should expect" more from their partners. The people in this category are promised more but given less and refuse to fight for what they deserve. The partners of these people are quite capable of giving more but they learn that they can get away with less. The following individual has unrealistically low expectations:

Sam was a middle-aged gay man married to David, who he met in college. While Sam and David initially agreed to have a monogamous relationship, David changed his mind three years into the marriage and demanded that the couple convert their relationship into a polyamorous one. Sam did not want to open his marriage to polyamory but feared disappointing

David. As a compromise to the double-bind he felt David had put him in, Sam suggested that the couple practice swinging rather than polyamory. This, he said, made him feel safer. But David refused and insisted that he desired a "special lover." Sam finally agreed to the new arrangement but given the way his relationship started out he clearly settled for less.

Notice in the previous cases that the individual with high realistic expectations, Keith, viewed his situation and his partner, Amanda, from a rational perspective. He knew what he wanted and what the odds were of getting it from her. There was little fantasy involved, and he used evidence and experience to support his expectations. He noticed cues and was less likely to repress his desires or to deny reality; he had greater ego strength. Specifically, Keith knew he was catered to by women, and that he adored them. He was also cognizant that because of his formidable experiences, he expected as much from Amanda but knew not to be overly demanding or expect all his needs to be unconditionally met.

The same can be said for the individual with realistically low expectations, Joyce. For example, Joyce knew that to keep her husband Alex, she had to give up her dream of having children. Although her realization was depressing to her, she justifiably accepted her evaluation of her situation and expected no more from it than it offered.

The person with unrealistically high expectations, Patty, was less likely to recognize "red flags," signaling that she would not get her expectations met. She was reluctant to openly express herself and when she did, she was vulnerable to being gaslighted, shut down, or abandoned. She tended to use fantasy to remain stuck in unfulfilling situations and made frequent use of other defense mechanisms to cope with her situations, most notably denial and repression. Patty deluded herself that her boyfriend, Terry, would stop staring at other women once married him and began having regular sex with him. But Terry never did.

And the person with unrealistic low expectations, Sam, was insightful yet paralyzed by his sad situation. Sam reluctantly agreed to an open, polyamorous marriage with his partner, David, for fear of losing him. Sam chose to settle for less than he wanted, but he felt that he had no choice; given David's strong convictions about having a polyamorous marriage, Sam felt settling for less was the prudent decision.

Internal Conflict

Another counterintuitive aspect of expectations that adds to the concept's complexity is that all couples, even the highest functioning, have conflicts. But couples only have one major internalized conflict – referred to in previous writings as a master conflict (Betchen, 2010). There are several master conflicts (Betchen & Davidson, 2018), but a conflict related to expectations is defined as an internal duality in which one part of a person wants their needs met and the other part is uncomfortable having them met (i.e., *having expectations met vs. not having expectations met*).

When this conflict is in "balance," couples are said to vacillate between the two sides with neither side dominating for any great length of time. In Figure 1.3 the couple "agree" to live a frugal lifestyle; they are said to be balanced. Figure 1.4 shows a couple who disagree on living a frugal lifestyle; they are said to be unbalanced. When the master conflict is "unbalanced" for too long it must be rebalanced to eradicate or alleviate symptoms. The closer the partners are to the extreme ends of the continuum of expectations the more intense the conflict and the more problematic the symptoms. Usually, the conflict is lodged in the unconscious and thus beyond awareness. But an especially insightful individual may be aware of at least one side of the conflict.

When an individual is experiencing an intense conflict, each side of the conflict will take turns sabotaging the other, making it impossible for the individual to get his/her expectations met. Many people, however, are not in a constant state of turmoil. When a couple are balanced, their internal conflicts are working together, and their most important expectations are being met.

As I explain later, people match up with others who have the same conflict – in this case, a conflict with expectations (see Chapter 3, Mate Choice and

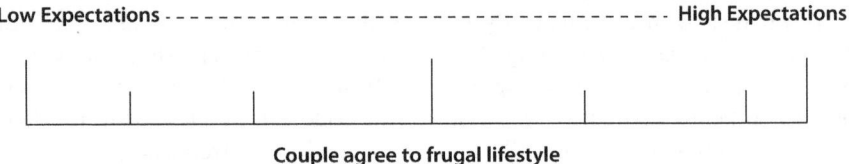

Low Expectations - High Expectations

Couple agree to frugal lifestyle

Figure 1.3   Balanced Expectations.

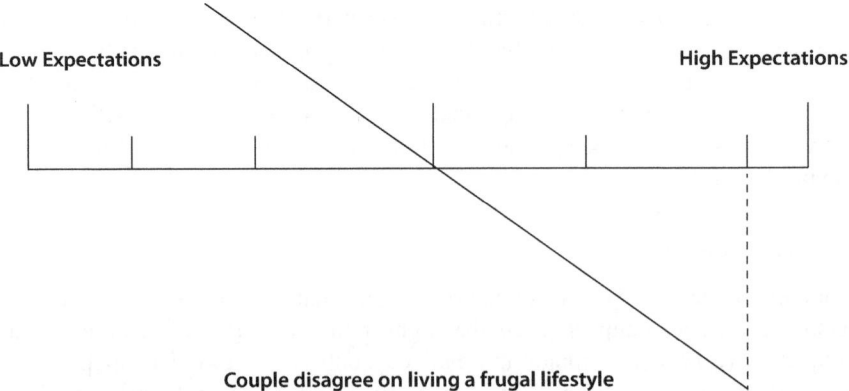

Low Expectations   High Expectations

Couple disagree on living a frugal lifestyle

Figure 1.4   Unbalanced Expectations.

Expectations). In a "shared conflict," the therapist must deal with both partners conspiring to maintain their conflict. This feat is especially difficult if the conflict is unbalanced because of a disagreement between the two partners concerning expectations.

Conflicts around expectations are impossible to fully eradicate because of the depth at which they exist. They are also difficult to manage, in part, because neither side of the conflict is necessarily right or wrong, making it difficult to choose one over the other. Choosing a side also results in change and change in turn can cause both anxiety and depression – the anxiety that comes with a new experience and the depression or sadness that comes with the loss of what is known. Gain and loss in this sense are associated with something that must be changed or given up in one's family of origin. For example, to meet your expectations you might have to lose the hatred you may be carrying for a parent or refuse to allow this hatred to interfere with your life's goals.

Rather than choose to suffer the anxiety that often comes with newness and the depression that may come with loss of the old, most individuals decide to live in the limbo of the conflict while trying to keep it under control as best they can. The goal of the therapist is to help each partner of a couple be able to: recognize and take responsibility of their conflict around expectations; understand the origin of their conflict; realize that the couple share the same conflict; integrate the two sides of the conflict with the use of differentiation in order to re-balance the conflict; and eradicate any associated nonsexual or sexual symptoms associated with the unbalanced conflict. These steps will be discussed in detail in the chapters ahead.

References

Baker, L., McNulty, J., & Vandergrift, L. (2017). Expectations for future relationship. *Experimental Psychology: General, 146*, 700–721. https://doi.org/10.1037/xge0000299

Beall, C. (2016). *Rebuilding a marriage better than new: Healing the broken places, resolving unmet expectations and moving your relationship forward.* Harvest House Publishers.

Betchen, S. (2010). *Magnetic partners: Discover how the hidden conflict that once attracted you to each other is now pulling you apart.* Free Press.

Betchen, S. (2022). *Couples in conflict: Navigating sexual and relationship control struggles in couples.* Routledge.

Betchen, S., & Davidson, H. (2018). *Master conflict therapy: A new model for practicing couples and sex therapy.* Routledge.

Betchen, S., & Gambescia, N. (2020). A new systemic treatment model for couples with premature ejaculation: Master Conflict Theory. In K. Hertlein, N. Gambescia, & G.Weeks (Eds.), *Systemic sex therapy* (3rd ed., pp. 77–91). Routledge.

Bian, T. (2021). 12 reasonable expectations that could save your marriage. Retrieved from www.divorcemag.com/blog/reasonable-expectations-save-your-marriage

Blair, S.L., & Madigan, T.J. (2016). Dating attitudes and expectations among young Chinese adults: an examination of gender differences. *The Journal of Chinese Sociology, 12*, 1–19. https://doi.org/10.1186/s40711-016-0034-1

Boszormenyi-Nagy, I., & Spark, G. (1973). *Invisible loyalties.* Harper & Row.

Casale, S., Fioravanti, G., Baldi, V., Flett, G., & Hewitt, P. (2019). Narcissism, perfectionistic self-presentation, and relationship satisfaction from a dyadic perspective. *Self and Identity*, 1–19. https://doi.org/10.1088/15298868.2019.1707272

Chapman, G. (2015). *The five love languages: The secret to love that lasts*. Northfield Publishing.

DiDonato, T. (2017, May). Expectations can hurt your relationships. Retrieved from www.psychologytoday.com/us/blog/meet-catch-and-keep/201705/expectations-can-hurt-your-relationship

Gambescia, N., Weeks, G., & Hertlein, K. (Eds.). (2021). *A clinician's guide to systemic sex therapy* (3rd ed.). Routledge.

Gottman, J., Silver, N. (2015). *The seven principles of marriage*. Harmony Books.

Grace, A. (2015). 12 common marriage expectations. Biola Center for Marriage & Relationships. Retrieved from https://cmr.biola.edu/blog/201

Harris, R. (2008). *The happiness trap: How to stop struggling and start living*. Trumpeter.

Hendrix, H., & Hunt, H.L. (2019). *Getting the love you want: A guide for couples*. St. Martin's Griffin.

Hertlein, K., Gambescia, N., & Weeks, N. (Eds.). (2020). *Systemic sex therapy* (3rd ed.). Routledge.

Johnson, S. (2019). *The practice of emotionally focused therapy* (3rd ed.). Routledge.

Kabra, P. (2019). Unmet expectations – The silent killer of all relationships. Retrieved from www.momspace.com/parenting/women-why-being-judged-always-article-unmet- expectations...

Khazan, O. (2017, September). We expect too much from our romantic partners. *The Atlantic*. Retrieved from www.the Atlantic.com/health/archive/2017/09/...

Kloppers, M. (2021). Unmet expectations thoughts on life and love. Retrieved from www.thoughtsonlove.com/unmet-expectations/1723/

National Fatherhood Initiative. (2005). With this ring... a national survey on marriage in America. Retrieved from www.fatherhood.org/with-this-ring-survey

Nelson, T. (Ed.). (2020). *Integrating couples and sex therapy*. PESI Publishing & Media.

Newbold. P. (2020). *Loved: A journal to bring joy to any marriage with dashed expectations and unmet needs*. Enjoy Being Married, LLC.

Perel, E. (2017). *Mating in captivity: Unlocking erotic intelligence*. Harper Paperbacks.

Vunnier, S.A., & O'Sullivan, L.F. (2018). Great expectations: Examining unmet romantic expectations and dating relationship outcomes using an investment model framework. *Journal of Social and Personal Relationships*, 35, 1045–1066. https://doi.org/10.1177/0265407517703492

2 The Origin of Expectations

It is quite normal to have expectations – everyone has them (Betchen, 2010). And it is equally normal to be disappointed from time to time – that's life. The primary interest of *Unmet Expectations* is how partners in a relationship process their expectations and handle their disappointments, and the specific relationship symptoms that may result. And to achieve this objective, it is important for each member of the couple to understand the "origin" of their expectations.

The Mother–Infant Bond

What starts out as a primitive instinctual need, with experience, develops into an expectation. From the time we are born we are dependent on our caregivers, especially the mother-figure, to satisfy our needs and for our very survival. If and how these needs are met often determines our expectations in life. Child theorists have long debated the idiosyncrasies of this special mother–infant bond albeit from different theoretical viewpoints. The following major psychoanalytic theories concerning the infant's needs and its relationship with the mother figure, at the very least, give people a starting point from which to think about how we develop expectations.

Sigmund Freud

Most theorists agreed that by 12 months of age, an infant develops a libidinal dependency on its mother-figure, but they did not all agree on the ways in which they came upon this dependency (Bowlby, 1958). Freud (1926/1959) claimed the infant is drawn primarily to the caregiver's breast that serves as the primary source of nourishment. It is only when the infant experiences that the breast is not always that available that it realizes that it is attached to the mother-figure. Thus, the actual bonding between mother and child forms in the second year of life when the baby makes this connection. According to Freud, because the child's prime concern is to satisfy a set of physiological needs, it is not yet concerned with establishing social connections. The child is in fact more anxious about the loss of the figure or object that meets these needs. Freud wrote:

DOI: 10.4324/9781003359470-3

But a moment's reflection takes us beyond this question of loss of object. The reason the infant in arms wants to perceive the presence of its mother is only because it already knows by experience that she satisfies all its needs without delay. The situation, then, which it regards as a "danger" and against which it wants to be safeguarded is that of nonsatisfaction, of a *growing tension due to need*, against which it is helpless.

(p. 137)

Freud also famously contended that the mother-figure simultaneously stimulates the child's erotic senses. "By her care of the child's body," he said "she becomes its first seducer. In these two relations lies the root of a mother's importance" (Freud, 1940/1964, p. 188). Freud saw this connection as the prototype for all later love-relations.

Bowlby (1958) referred to Freud's theory as one of *Secondary Drive* because social connection is secondary to or derived from primary drives like hunger. According to Bowlby (1969), "The secondary drive holds that a liking to be with other members of the species is a result of being fed by them" (p. 211).

Anna Freud

In 1941, Anna Freud and her partner and fellow child psychoanalyst Dorothy Burlingham opened the Hampstead War Nurseries – which they primarily formed to aid children traumatized by the London bombings in World War II. Financed by the Foster Parents' Plan for War Children, the nurseries included a large residential nursery for babies and young children; a day nursery for children from the residential nursery, and others; and a country house for evacuated London children ages 3–6. At these nurseries Freud and her colleagues were given the opportunity to observe children's interactions with and without their mothers from birth (Freud & Burlingham, 1942, 1943).

Several valuable publications came out of the work at the war nurseries, one being *Infants Without Families* (Freud & Burlingham, 1944). In this book the authors focused on the developmental process of infants in residential nurseries and their relationships with each other, and substitute caregivers. Comparisons were drawn between the care offered by parents versus the substitute care provided by the residential facilities. The authors wrote:

We have chosen four distinct aspects of the infant's life to illustrate the differences in development under home and institutional conditions: Muscular Control, Speech Development, Habit Training and Feeding. The differences in each case were quantitative: muscular control and good eating habits develop more quickly and easily in institutions; speech and habit training are delayed when the mother's influence is missing.

(p. 27)

At the war nurseries, Anna Freud herself focused specifically on children, from infants to toddlers, who were deprived of maternal care and those who were experiencing separation. In doing so she came to believe, as did Bowlby (1953, 1973) and Winnicott (1940/2017), in the caregiver's importance to young children, and the "consequences to broken attachments" (Midgley, 2007, p. 946). Some of the symptoms she noted were anxiety, increased aggression, guilt thinking that they caused their own abandonment, and regressive behavior such as enuresis and thumb sucking. Freud and Burlingham (1943) admitted the wartime dilemma that children and workers faced at the nurseries: The children either stay home and experience death and destruction of war and the associated anxiety of their mothers, or they enter a nursery and experience maternal separation. "Choosing between two evils seems to be all that war-time care is able to accomplish for them" (p. 84).

Despite her countless observations and findings, however, Anna Freud never abandoned her father's drive theory. She wrote:

> … that the relationship to the mother, although the first to another human being, is not infant's first relationship to the environment. What precedes it is an earlier phase in which not the object world, but the body needs, and their satisfaction or frustration play the decisive part.
>
> (Freud, 1954, p. 321)

She went on to say:

> At the beginning of life, the infant organism is governed by the vital body needs for respiration, sleep, intake of food, evacuation, skin comfort, and movement, which are the forerunners and first representatives of the basic drives.
>
> (Freud, 1954, p. 322)

Melanie Klein

Melanie Klein (1952/2018) emphasized the importance of interpersonal relationships (e.g., closeness and nurturing from the mother-figure) over biologically based drives in her theory of object relations. She believed that the relationship between infants and caregivers is said to serve as a prototype for future relationships. Klein wrote:

> Some children who, although good feeders, are not markedly greedy, show unmistakable signs of love and of a developing interest in the mother at an early stage – an attitude which contains some of the essential elements of an object-relation.
>
> (p. 96)

From birth, Klein felt that ego formation began in the infant's unconscious "phantasy" world by relating to the world through part-objects. To illustrate, the primary object-mother becomes the part-object breast. The infant looks to the breast for nourishment and security. When the mother-figure is available and provides this for the infant, the infant is satisfied and has loving feelings towards the object-breast. In this sense, the infant has positive feelings towards what it perceives as a dependable, and secure provider of its needs. The mother's breast, however, is not always available, and this frustrates the infant who in turn feels anxious and persecuted. This creates negative feelings such as hate towards the object-breast.

Klein believed that the young ego had little capacity to tolerate anxiety (Klein, 1932/2018). To protect both the infant and the ego from the anxiety associated with the two contradictory feelings of love and hate provoked by the inconsistencies of nurturing (as well as the birth trauma and the ever present fear of annihilation by the inherent death instinct; Klein, 1946/2018), the infant "splits" the object-breast, and "projects" separately its loving and hating feelings (life and death instincts) into separate parts of the same mother (i.e., breasts); the result being "good breast" (i.e., loved, nourishing breast) and "bad breast" (i.e., hated, persecutory, withholding breast).

The infant then projects and introjects the good and bad breasts. The infant projects their bad qualities such as hate outwards, into the bad breast, and introjects or takes in the good objects such as love, from the good breast. The infant can then make a clear distinction between the "good objects," which are now inside them, and the "bad objects," which have been split from them.

Klein (1946/2018) believed that splitting was important to healthy development. She wrote: "the process of splitting off parts of the self and projecting them into objects are thus of vital importance for normal developments as well as for normal object-relations" (p. 9). This developmental stage occurs from birth up to four or six months and is what Klein (1946/2018) called the *paranoid-schizoid position.*

When the infant comes to realize that the mother-object in total is not only responsible for meeting its needs but frustrating them as well (i.e., the mother is both good and bad), the mother is seen as whole. The infant must then deal with the guilt for having attacked the good object during the *paranoid schizoid position*, and cope with the fear of losing both the idealized good object and a part of the self. An ardent desire for reparation is also evident. In this position, the ego is integrated and strengthened, and omnipotent control over the object becomes more realistic, although according to Klein (1963/2018): "Full and permanent integration is never possible for some polarity between the life and death instincts always persists and remains the deepest source of conflict" (p. 302). Klein (1935/2018) called this stage – from the middle to the first year of life – the *depressive position.* Given that the Kleinian model is based heavily on the infant's reliance on the mother's breast, oral cravings are dominant in her theory.

Donald Winnicott

Winnicott proposed a humanistic, personal connection between mother and infant from the birth of the infant. He claimed that maternal care has a profound impact on the development of the child. According to Winnicott, mother and infant are one in the infant's mind. He wrote: "At the beginning, by an almost 100% adaptation affords the infant the opportunity for the illusion that her breast is part of the infant" (Winnicott, 1971/2005, p. 15). While it is necessary that the onset for the infant's "transitory object" be the mother's breast, the goal of the maternal/infant relationship is always to help the infant to gradually move from this dependent state towards one of functional autonomy. In Winnicott's words: "The mother who is able to give herself over, for a limited spell, to this her natural task, is able to protect her infant's *going-on-being*" (Winnicott, 1963/2017, p. 472).

Winnicott believed it was primarily up to the mother to provide an environment to help the infant transition through various developmental stages towards independence. To facilitate this process, the mother creates what Winnicott calls a "holding environment." Holding includes much more than the physical holding of the infant but includes "the whole routine of care throughout the day and night, and it is not the same with any two infants because it is a part of the infant, and no two infants are alike. Also, it follows the minute day-to-day changes belonging to the infant's growth and development, both physical and psychological" (Winnicott, 1965/2018, p. 49). Winnicott claimed that during the maternal/infant stage what is happening outside of the infant's body, in its environment of care, impacts the individual's later expectations of others and the world – much of which is determined by the mother-figure's ability to create a good holding environment.

Winnicott used the term "good enough mother" to depict a mother that was not a "perfect" parent – in fact, he saw this as potentially detrimental to the child – but one that was attentive, empathic, and conscientious enough to meet the particular or idiosyncratic needs of "her infant," both physiological and psychological. If the mother was a "good enough" caregiver, the child had a much better chance of developing a "true self" or a more authentic person true to their own feelings and value – an individual with a strong ego. In Winnicott's words: "The good enough mother meets the omnipotence of the infant and makes sense of it. She does this repeatedly. A true self begins to have life through the strength given to the infant's weak ego by the mother's implementation of the infant's omnipotent expressions" (Winnicott, 1965/2018, p. 145). In his book *Playing and Reality*, Winnicott (1971/2005) claimed that a true self is the only self that can be creative, and that "playing" helps in this development.

In contrast, if the mother-figure is a "not good enough mother," she is not good enough "to implement the infant's omnipotence, and so she repeatedly fails to meet the infant gesture; instead, she substitutes her own gesture which is to be given sense by the compliance of the infant" (Winnicott, 1965/2018, p. 145).

Simply put, rather than meet her baby's specific needs, this mother enables the baby to adapt to her needs and desires. In this case, the child develops a "false self" or one who adapts to or follows all rules regardless of their true feelings; the ego remains underdeveloped (Winnicott, 1964/2017).

Bowlby (1958) contended that Winnicott's ideas do not neatly fit into his proposed theoretical categories of *Secondary Drive, Primary Object Sucking, Primary Object Clinging,* or *Return-to-Womb Craving.* As noted, Winnicott's theory is both humanistic and intimate in nature. Although a psychoanalyst, Winnicott was also a pediatrician – this may in part be responsible for his specific developmental approach to mother and child, and any associated expectations.

John Bowlby

Rejecting the theory of *Secondary Drive,* Bowlby (1958) combines *Primary Object Sucking* and *Primary Object Clinging* theories to suggest that the infant has a natural need to both suck on a human breast and cling to a human, meaning the mother-figure. He did not exclude the need for physiological drive but found that there is also an inherent need for an object that is independent of food; one based on social contact.

Bowlby (1969) was heavily influenced by the experiments of Lorenz (1935), who found that newly hatched baby ducklings and goslings would follow any moving object or person without being reinforced by food, and in time will favor the object over all others. This learning process became famously known as "imprinting."

Harry Harlow's work with Rhesus monkeys also influenced Bowlby (1969). Immediately following birth, infant monkeys were separated from their mothers and placed in cages with surrogate mother-figures made of wood and wire; others were covered in soft terrycloth. Despite the wire surrogates having milk to offer, the infant monkeys preferred the softer surrogates made of terrycloth, except when hungry (Harlow & Zimmerman, 1958). Harlow (1961) wrote:

> When the cloth mother was present, the infant would rush wildly to her, climb upon her, rub against her, and cling to her tightly… However, when the cloth mother was absent, the infants would rush across the test room and threw themselves face downward, clutching their heads and bodies and screaming their distress…
>
> (p. 78)

When the cloth mother was present in the infant monkeys' immediate environment (i.e., cage), they also felt secure enough to explore their surroundings. Bowlby (1969,1973, 1980) studied the distress infants experience when separated from the mother-figure and found similar reactions at separation (i.e., crying, screaming).

Bowlby (1969, 1973) claimed that a child looks to the mother-figure for consistent empathic responses for comfort and support. If this is the case, the child's worthiness is reinforced, and they develop a secure attachment style. If the mother-figure has been inconsistent, the attachment to the caregiver will be insecure and lead to insecure attachment style. He contended that continual disruption of the attachment between infant and primary mother-figure could result in long-term cognitive, social, and emotional difficulties for that infant. Bowlby believed that the earliest bonds formed by children with their first caregivers have a tremendous impact that continues throughout life.

The Family of Origin

While psychoanalysts look to the mother–infant bond as the origin of our early and later life expectations, many systemic therapists, especially those practicing psychodynamic work, attribute these expectations to each person's family of origin. In doing so, they may not look as far back as analysts to determine the origin of expectations but work with whatever information the individual consciously provides or unconsciously reveals and then applies this information to their current situation. This enables both individual and therapist to see a direct connection between family of origin influences and their expectations.

As mentioned in Chapter 1, Introduction: Complexity and Conflict, I apply the MCT model to couples with symptoms related to expectations in their relationships (Betchen, 2010, 2017; Betchen & Davidson, 2018; Betchen & Gambescia, 2020). MCT teaches that unconscious conflicts influenced by each partners' families of origin are responsible for the degree and intensity of their expectations. Whether these reactions are realistic or unrealistic, their respective histories offer an alibi for their behavior. In this sense, there is a reason for everything. The conflicts reside in all of us, and we cannot help but bring them to our relationships. The following are some of the ways in which someone can develop an internal conflict with expectations that can impact their later relationships.

Indulged/Spoiled

If you were indulged as a child and your every desire fulfilled by at least one parent, you can grow up feeling entitled to having your expectations met. In adult relationships, you might then expect to be catered to and see nothing wrong with being in a one-sided relationship in which your partner consistently sacrifices for you. Working hard to keep your partner happy may be a foreign concept to you, in part because having your own needs met has always been the priority. If you were the youngest of older siblings, especially the youngest brother of sisters or the youngest sister of brothers, you were more likely to get your needs met. Toman (1976) wrote:

> The youngest brother of sisters is a great one with the ladies. They love him and are anxious to care for him. They want to keep house for him, to handle his files or his suits. To cook for him, etc.
>
> (p. 163)

> Being the first and only male among his siblings, he has usually been allowed to do or refuse to do more than others were. He has little competition. His sisters were expected to protect and serve him. Inadvertently and partly unconsciously he worked this situation to his advantage. He is not likely to forgo his privileges in life and at work if he can help it.
>
> (p. 164)

> He needs a kind, warm, and motherly person who is ready to overlook his flaws and keeps a skillful and supportive hand in his affairs.
>
> (p. 165)

Of the youngest sister of brothers, Toman (1976) said:

> She is a good friend, willing to apply and devote herself if a person whom she loves requests it. She also gets what she wants from men. Sometimes she seems a bit spoiled or even extravagant.
>
> (p. 181)

In some families of origin, the most prized child in a family might turn out to be the oldest, especially if they are longed-for, the most competent, or particularly talented. A female client told me that she had six miscarriages until having her first child, a girl. And this was to remain her special child for life. Another told me what her mother-in-law said about her first child, a boy: "Thank God that it was a boy. Now we can open a bottle of champagne." The boy was eventually nicknamed "the little prince," and was treated like royalty well into adulthood.

If not in conflict, the indulged individual will choose someone, as Toman (1976) mentioned, who prefers to be a caretaker and the match will be a complementary one with little to no issues. If, however, this type of individual is in conflict about getting needs met out of guilt, for example, he/she may simultaneously block or sabotage this from happening. The following is an example of this conflict in action:

Kent was the oldest child of two brothers; his parents could not wait to have him. Kent claimed that his upbringing was a dream and that he loved his parents dearly. He grew up with a wonderful sense of self-esteem and self-worth and did well at every endeavor. He was handsome and a fine athlete, and he always had plenty of friends. And while Kent appreciated his success, he was in emotional conflict that at times blocked him from achieving even greater heights.

Kent got into several prestigious colleges that were willing to give him money to attend. But he chose a school of lesser stature and took a part-time job to pay for his education. His parents were confused by some of his decisions. Kent also turned down numerous honors in high school and college claiming that it was better to be humble.

Kent reported for treatment because he had recently had a fight with his boss that cost him a promotion and a large salary increase. He said that it seemed to come out of nowhere. "I just exploded," he said. "My boss has always been great to me. He gave me everything I ever wanted and has mentored me up the ladder at the company." Kent also claimed that he has been feeling noticeably depressed for some time.

Kent's family of origin revealed that he had a younger brother who suffered from a developmental disability that made it difficult for him to achieve Kent's status. Because of this, Kent claimed that while he loved the accolades that his parents and others heaped upon him, he felt guilty receiving them. He said that the more accolades the greater the guilt.

Kent wanted his younger brother to succeed but despite doing all he could for him, it was never going to be enough. Kent wanted his needs met, but he also sabotaged them at times just to maintain a certain emotional balance with his conflict. If Kent's brother would have achieved a modicum of success Kent might have been able to avoid this conflict, but it was not to be.

Abused/Neglected

Children who have been abused or neglected may feel they have paid their dues in childhood. As adults they may then feel entitled to have their expectations met and react strongly when they are denied. Some may even experience a post-traumatic reaction when they are denied. The other side of this, however, is that because they were mistreated by those who were supposed to love them unconditionally, they internalize feelings of low self-worth and with it a question as to whether they are deserving or not. Thus, on the one hand they feel they are entitled and on the other hand they are not sure they deserve to be. The following case illustrates this conflict:

Janice was abandoned by her father at age four and physically and verbally abused by her alcoholic mother thereafter. Blessed with good looks and natural intelligence Janice was popular in high school and graduated without much effort. Few of her friends knew what life was really like for

Janice and saw her as someone with high self-esteem who was justified in having her needs met by friends, boyfriends, and even teachers in her school.

Because of her beauty, Janice was able to attract many boys and in fact, married one of them soon out of high school. The boy she chose was smart, handsome and from a nice, intact family with money. This young man worshipped Janice. He could not believe he landed the diva of their high school and Janice contributed to this myth. She expected him to cater to her and could be quite abusive if he failed to live up to her standards.

While Janice's new husband and his family made sure she had everything she could ever want, without any apparent provocation Janice made the decision to have an affair with a local car mechanic with whom she got pregnant. Despite having an abortion and leaving her lover once this was exposed in the community, Janice's husband and his family abandoned and disgraced Janice. Faced with having to relocate, Janice's once idyllic lifestyle was destroyed, and her reputation would never recover in her hometown. Even with some alimony Janice eventually had to take welfare and food stamps to survive. In treatment Janice said with some insight: "I guess I ended up where I started from. I got exactly what I felt I deserved."

Mixed Messages

A conflict with expectations can also develop if one parent or parents give mixed verbal messages about what you deserve. For example, your parents may tell you that you are brilliant your entire life. But when it comes to sending you to college, they may find an excuse not to. In this sense there is a double message: you are smart but not smart enough to support. In some families each parent might send a message that contradicts the others. For example, one parent might say: "I believe in you so I will help you" while the other might tell you: "I don't think you've got what it takes so I will not invest in you."

Some parents convey contradictory mixed verbal/physical messages which can negatively impact a child's ability to be intimate as an adult. For example, a parent might consistently tell you how much they love you but fail to hug or kiss you even at the most appropriate times. This leaves the child confused, not knowing what they should or should not expect from others. Many clients have told me that they knew that their parents loved them, but they have no real emotional or physical proof of this. Consider Michael's case:

Michael's mother and father fought constantly. His father accused his mother of being too demanding and infantile and his mother accused his father of infidelity and ruining the family business. Because Michael's father treated him as if he were a burden, Michael grew close to his mother and together they formed a coalition against his father.

Throughout Michael's life his mother always stood up for him and told him he was the greatest. She defended him against any of his critics including demanding teachers, family members, and especially his father. Michael's father on the other hand consistently criticized Michael and treated him as if he were a burden. He would never give Michael the satisfaction of pleasing him.

As Michael grew up, he expected everyone to treat him as his mother did even if he was in the wrong or did little to earn their respect. However, on a deeper level Michael felt like a fraud and was shocked when people met or exceeded his expectations. In this sense, there existed a deep shame that contributed to his conflict with expectations courtesy of his father.

Broken Promises

Like mixed messages but different enough to merit its own subsection, some parents make a promise to a child but never had any intention to keep it; others could not keep their promise because of unforeseen circumstances. The latter is far more excusable because life has its many twists and turns. But when a promise is made in good faith and there is no just reason to fail to keep it, a child may develop a conflict around expectations. Again, if you cannot trust your parents who can you trust? Consider Gerry's case:

Gerry reported for treatment both angry and anxious. He told me that all his life his parents were insistent that he had to go to college. Wanting to please them, Gerry tried his hardest and was accepted to several competitive but reasonable expensive schools. After Gerry decided on a school, and one that his parents approved of, they told him to take out as many school loans as he could and when it came time to pay the loans back, they would take responsibility. Thinking that his parents were trying to teach him a life lesson he obliged and got himself into great debt. Following graduation, however, when Gerry approached his parents for financial help his father told him that he did not have the money and that Gerry should get a job as soon as possible.

Gerry expected his parents to fulfill their promise and could not comprehend that they would do such a thing to him, especially since their financial position did not deteriorate in the last four years. He said: "I cannot believe that my parents did that to me. I could never trick my own children like that and risk them distrusting me the rest of their lives."

Traumatic Events

Sometimes a conflict with expectations can emerge from a traumatic experience. Some people have told me they feel cursed because of something tragic happening to them. One response to this was to adopt a nihilistic stance and rid themselves of all positive expectations. These individuals are always "waiting for the other shoe to drop." If they happen to feel personally responsible for the tragedy, they may want to pardon themselves but feel far too guilty to do so. This is evident in cases of "survivor guilt."

Todd's mother died of a heart attack on his wedding day. Shocked and suffering from tremendous guilt, Todd blamed himself because he married a woman of whom she didn't approve. Nevertheless, when Todd's honeymoon trip was marred by horrible weather, Todd, already feeling guilty, said that he felt cursed as well. He said that while he wanted to live a good life with his new wife, he expected the worst to happen to them at any given time, and that they deserved it.

Siblings with Different Expectations

It is possible to grow up in the same family and yet have different expectations in adulthood. For example, a brother, Ari, and sister, Hannah, were raised in a Jewish household run by perfectionistic and hypercritical parents. And while Ari became a lawyer and Hannah became an accountant, Ari – now a man with a family, was incredibly angry with his parents and has maintained his distance.

Ari eventually married an overly critical and demanding woman who he was on the verge of divorcing. When questioned why he married this woman Ari said that he initially thought she was supportive and would understand his position with his parents. Instead, however, she often sided with them in arguments and insisted that it was important her children have regular access to their grandparents. She expected this much from the family she married into.

On the contrary, Hannah has remained close to her parents and never married. She said that she expected little from marriage and that she would rather have control over her life. Hannah went on to blame a terrible experience with a former "controlling" boyfriend for this attitude. Oddly, when Ari and Hannah communicated, it was as if they had completely different experiences or come from two different families, and yet they were only two years apart in age. Ari tried to tell Hannah that the parents were responsible for her attitude towards marriage. Hannah vehemently disagreed and said that he, not their parents, were the cause of his impending divorce.

While it is possible that only one sibling can develop a problematic conflict with expectations, it is highly unlikely. Even though Ari and Hannah had vastly different perceptions of their parents, the parents' hypercritical behavior was responsible for their different but equally troublesome expectations in adulthood. When the family of origin produces a master conflict, no one escapes it; it merely shows up in different forms and contexts.

There are several different ways to think about the origin of expectations from the psychoanalytic to the systemic, and they all give a glimpse into the importance of the role that our pasts play in this developmental process. While the MCT model borrows from others, it never wavers from considering the importance of the family of origin's role in the shaping of and reaction to our expectations, met and unmet. The next chapter will focus on the role that conflicts with expectations play in our attraction and mate choice.

References

Betchen, S. (2010). *Magnetic partners: Discover how the hidden conflict that once attracted you to each other is now pulling you apart*. Free Press.

Betchen, S. (2022). *Couples in conflict: Navigating sexual and relationship control struggles in couples*. Routledge.

Betchen, S., & Davidson, H. (2018). *Master conflict therapy: A new model for practicing couples and sex therapy*. Routledge.

Betchen, S., & Gambescia, N. (2020). A new systemic treatment model for couples with premature ejaculation: Master Conflict Theory. In K. Hertlein, N. Gambescia, & G. Weeks (Eds.), *Systemic sex therapy* (3rd ed., pp. 77–91). Routledge.

Bowlby, J. (1953). Some pathological processes set in train by early mother-child separation. *Journal of Mental Science, 99*, 265–272.

Bowlby, J. (1958). The nature of the child's tie to his mother. *International Journal of Psychanalysis, 39*, 350–373.

Bowlby, J. (1969). *Attachment and loss: Vol. 1. Attachment* (2nd ed.). Basic Books.

Bowlby, J. (1973). *Attachment and loss: Vol. 2. Separation: Anxiety and anger* (2nd ed.). Basic Books.

Bowlby, J. (1980). *Attachment and loss: Vol. 3. Loss: Sadness and depression* (2nd ed.). Basic Books

Freud, A. (1954). Psycho-analysis and education. In A. Freud (Ed.), *The writings of Anna Freud: Indications for child analysis and other papers* (Vol. IV, pp. 317–326). International Universities Press.

Freud, A., & Burlingham, D. (1942). *Young children in war time: A year's work in a residential war nursery*. George Allen & Unwin.

Freud, A., & Burlingham, D. (1943). *War and children*. Medical War Books.

Freud, A., & Burlingham, D. (1944). *Infants without families*. Medical War Books and International University Press.

Freud, S. (1926/1959). Inhibitions, symptoms and anxiety. In J. Strachey (Ed. and Trans.), *The standard edition of the complete psychological works of Sigmund Freud* (Vol. 20, pp. 87–175). Hogarth Press and the Institute for Psychoanalysis.

Freud, S. (1940/1964). An example of psycho-analytic work. In J. Strachey (Ed. and Trans.), *The standard edition of the complete psychological works of Sigmund Freud* (Vol. 23, pp. 183–194). Hogarth Press and the Institute for Psychoanalysis.

Harlow, H. F. (1961). The development of affectional patterns in infant monkeys.' In B. M. Foss (Ed.), *Determinants of Infant Behaviour I* (pp. 75–88). Methuen & Co., LTD.

Harlow, H. F., & Zimmermann, R.R. (1958). The development of affective responsiveness in infant monkeys. *Proceedings of the American Philosophical Society*, *102*, 501–509.

Klein, M. (1932/2018). An observational neurosis in a 6-year-old girl. In M. Klein (Ed.), *The collected works of Melanie Klein: The psycho-analysis of children.* (Vol. II, pp. 35–57). Routledge.

Klein, M. (1935/2018). A contribution to the psychogenesis of manic-depressive states. In M. Klein (Ed.), T*he collected works of Melanie Klein: "Love, guilt and reparation" and other works 1921–1945.* (Vol I. pp. 262–289). Routledge.

Klein, M. (1946/2018). Notes on some schizoid mechanisms. In M. Klein (Ed.), *The collected works of Melanie Klein: "Envy and gratitude" and other works* 1946–1963. (Vol. III, pp. 1–24). Routledge.

Klein, M. (1952/2018). On observing the behaviour of young infants. In M. Klein (Ed.), *The collected works of Melanie Klein: "Envy and gratitude" and other works* 1946–1963. (Vol. III, pp. 91–121). Routledge.

Klein, M. (1963/2018). On the sense of loneliness. In M. Klein (Ed.), T*he collected works of Melanie Klein: "Envy and gratitude" and other works 1946–1963.* (Vol III. pp. 300–313). Routledge.

Lorenz, K. (1935). Der Kumpan in der Umwelt des Vogels. *Journal of Ornithologie*, *83*, 137–213. https://doi.org/10.1007/BF01905355

Midgley, N. (2007). Anna Freud: The Hampstead War Nurseries and the role of the direct observation of children for psychoanalysis. *International Journal of Psycho-Analysis*, *88*, 939–959.

Toman, W. (1976). *Family constellation: Its effects on personality and social behavior.* Springer.

Winnicott, D. W. (1940/2017). Children and their mothers. In L. Caldwell & H.T. Robinson (Eds.), *The collected works of D.W. Winnicott* (Vol. 2, pp. 81–86). Oxford University Press.

Winnicott, D. W. (1963/2017). From dependence towards independence in the development of the individual. In L. Caldwell & H.T. Robinson (Eds.), *The collected works of D.W. Winnicott* (Vol. 6, pp. 469–477). Oxford University Press.

Winnicott, D. W. (1964/2017). The concept of the false self. In L. Caldwell & H.T. Robinson (Eds.), *The collected works of D.W. Winnicott* (Vol. 7, pp. 27–31). Oxford University Press.

Winnicott, D. W. (1965/2018). *The maturational processes and the facilitating environment.* Routledge.

Winnicott, D. W. (1971/2005). *Playing and reality.* Routledge.

3   Mate Choice and Expectations

As mentioned in Chapter 1, Introduction: Complexity and Conflict, people unconsciously choose a mate with the same conflict. In previous writings they were referred to as "twins-in-conflict" (Betchen, 2010; Betchen, 2022; Betchen & Davidson, 2018). In this context, one mate chooses another with the same internalized conflict with expectations (i.e., *having expectations met vs. not having expectations met*).

By choosing someone with the same conflict, a newly formed couple can almost guarantee that their shared conflict will prove to be a formidable defense against the discomfort that change brings, be it anxiety or depression. In support of this, a male client scared of change commented: "I'd rather stick with the devil I know rather than the devil I don't know."

Couples who collude in this type of defensive system are quite challenging and often place the couples therapist in a double bind: "Make our symptoms disappear but do not change us." Another way of interpreting this might be: "Get rid of our pain but without the change." In my clinical experience, most people do not seem to mind change if they are "guaranteed" that it will be painless and will work to their advantage, something the clinician cannot and should not promise.

When a couple share a conflict, they specifically protect themselves from change with a sophisticated process: pulling each other back whenever one leans towards one side of the conflict over the other. In the context of expectations, if one partner begins to feel primarily deserved or entitled the other partner will let them know that they are not in fact as worthy as they might think. If, on the other hand, the same partner swings towards the other side of the conflict and feels they are never deserved of anything, the partner will give them a boost and let them know that this is not true; that they are worth or entitled to more than they think. This process is mostly unconscious and therefore easy for each partner to avoid taking responsibility.

Janice felt that her husband Scott was being taken advantage of by the company he had worked at for 25 years. She expected him to stand up for himself and said that he needed to "be a man." It was true that Scott had received few raises and no promotions even though he had always performed to his company's standards. But when he finally got the courage to demand a raise, he

DOI: 10.4324/9781003359470-4

was immediately terminated for what his boss called "disloyalty." Janice then blamed Scott for what she said was his "stupidity and short-sightedness." Scott was able to tolerate his wife's response because he was conflicted about what he should expect of himself and others.

Terri, who was an only child, expected that she would be the center of her husband Richard's universe, even though it also embarrassed her. However, Richard came from a large, close-knit family in which no one person stood out. While he paid equal attention to Terri, he expected her to cooperate and fit right in with his family, as if she were one of the cogs in a giant wheel. But he also would get a little tired of his family's relentless social requirements.

Each partner takes turns throughout the life of a couple balancing and re-balancing the conflict so that it stays stable. If, for example one partner of a middle-class family happens upon a financial windfall, to maintain conflict balance, either he/she will feel guilty about it or find a way to get rid of it. As a failsafe, the other partner might sabotage the winnings somehow. Symptoms develop when the conflict is out of balance for too long a time. This might mean that one partner changes or grows enough and is less conflicted.

Janie was a low-level employee in a human resource department who expected little of herself professionally, and rarely complained about her plight. However, once her company went public Janie became rich, something she never expected in her wildest dreams. Her husband Ted, on the other hand, worked for a school system and constantly complained about being underpaid. He believed that as a college-educated man he should have been better compensated. While it would only be logical that once the couple struck it rich, all would be well. This might raise Janie's self-esteem and satisfy Ted's need for financial justice. However, Ted began to criticize Janie for getting something she did not deserve, and Janie slipped into a guilt-ridden depression.

While the conflicts may have been caused by different circumstances, the result is the same – a conflict with expectations. For example, consider the case of Jim and Marcia. Jim developed his expectations from being infantilized by an over-protective mother. She was always defending him, right or wrong, against outsiders, and against his critical father. But she was also intrusive when it came to his love life and got into skirmishes with several of his girlfriends whom she found never to be good enough for her son. As a result, Jim expected to be treated like he was special by the women in his life, especially his wife Marcia, but at times he would feel angrily smothered by it. Marcia developed her expectations from being neglected by her parents. She felt she was owed attention, and less likely to shower Jim with it, but did so angrily out of fear he would find a better caregiver and replace her. Jim and Marcia's conflicts with expectations originated from opposite experiences but each partner still developed a conflict with expectations.

It is impossible according to conflict theory for someone to choose a mate with a different conflict. Even with sufficient insight – which few people have – the best one can do is to choose someone with the same conflict who has more conscious control over it so that the conflict will not be so easily unbalanced.

The attraction to someone with the same conflict is magnetic (Betchen, 2010). Clients and friends as well have told me that they will wait until they have found the perfect person for them. I hear this especially from those people who have had a bad or traumatic experience with a long-term relationship. I empathize with the sentiment. However, this strategy will not protect them from another relationship disaster. Without insight, time will be of no value. The underlying conflict is very patient. It will wait for us to choose someone with the same conflict... again. Consider Stuart and Julia:

Stuart had been in a miserable, sexless marriage for 19 years. When he finally got the courage to divorce, he pledged to his friends that he would purposely stay single until he found a more loving woman. True to his word, Stuart got an apartment with an old college friend and led the single life for nine years. Stuart was proud of dating so many women at this time in his life, but one day he met Julia.

Julia was a sexy, never-married woman who met all of Stuart's needs. Thinking that he had waited long enough, and sure of his choice, Stuart quickly married Julia. But within six months of marriage Julia decided to find religion and give up sex. She said that she had been promiscuous as a young woman and now that she is married, she will make up for her sins with celibacy. Stuart could not believe that he had waited nine years only to make the same mistake. In truth Stuart did not mind Julia's past adventures. He took them as solid evidence that he could expect a robust sex life. He then spent many years trying to change Julia but with limited success.

While I consider choosing a long-term partner primarily an unconscious, deterministic process, I do believe that physical attraction plays a role in mate selection. In fact, I believe that each partner chooses someone that they are physically attracted to, but an individual with the same master conflict. If, for example, someone is attracted to tall blond-haired people, this will influence who they choose for a mate, but for the relationship to take hold, the tall blond-haired person chosen must also possess the same conflict.

Conflict theory does not apply to flings, only to long-term commitments. Anyone can take a rest from a conflict and have sex with someone they find purely physically attractive. However, this type of relationship will not last. Each will eventually choose to match up with someone with the same conflict. This might explain why a man, for example, might exclusively date blonde women with a certain body type, but shock his friends and family when he chooses to settle down with a brown-haired person with an entirely different body type. People often think that the unexpected shift is a sign of phoniness when in fact the phoniness was in the dating process.

Jan told me in treatment that she was surprised at herself for marrying a short man. "Although I would complain about dating tall men because kissing them bothered my neck, that's all I ever dated. Then I go and marry a short man. I do not get it." With examination, Jan felt taller men could better protect her and fit better into society's stereotype that men should be taller than the women they date and *vice versa*. But because these men failed to have the same underlying conflict with expectations, Jan found a shorter man who did. In this sense, looks count but are usually sacrificed in the service of the conflict.

It is also conceivable that our conflicts shape physical attraction to a certain extent. That is, you may think your choice of mate fits your physical requirements when it is the underlying conflict that is the motivating factor in your choice. I am sure you have heard some people comment: "They don't look like a match." Or something like: "She is way out of his league." To the outside observer this is stating the obvious, but no matter how stark the difference in physical attraction may be, you can be sure the conflicts are the same. The partners are closer to being the same than meets the eye. I have said many times that in all the years I have worked with couples, I have never seen a bad match. I have seen destructive matches but never mismatches.

While MCT is a deterministic model, it helps to explain why people will stay with each other even in some of the darkest times. And it also explains why they tend to remarry the same type of person over and over. I believe that the divorce rate for second marriages is so high: approximately 60%, up from 50% for first marriages (World Population Review, 2022) in part, because we unconsciously choose the same partner again. And when we expect more and better, we get the same.

It is sad to see people who are so consciously looking forward to a better life, only to remarry into the same dynamic. Even affairs usually do not work very well because people have them with those who share the same conflict as their spouses. And the rates of divorce for marrying your lover are even higher: approximately 73% (World Population Review, 2022). But it is a tricky process because while in an affair, you are usually arguing with your spouse or bringing out the worst in one another. The lover has the advantage of telling you how wonderful you are and that you deserve better. But if you deserve better, why would you put yourself through the same thing again?

To gain control over a conflict, some people take a purely behavioral approach, and this is a common mistake. For example, rather than deal with his unrealistic expectations of marriage, Larry married and divorced five times. Larry thought that he was simply marrying the wrong woman and all he needed to do was to find the right one. But Larry's approach was unique. He insisted on marrying women of different races and religions all the while expecting a different outcome. Considering himself Catholic, he first married a nice Catholic girl from his neighborhood. When that relationship failed, he married a Protestant woman. When that marriage failed, Larry married a Jewish woman. But when that relationship failed, Larry decided to take the international route and married what he thought was an obedient, Japanese woman. Instead, she turned out to be less compliant than Larry expected, and he divorced again. He then married his fifth wife, a Hindu. Regardless of the variety, because Larry refused to examine his internal issues, they all ended the same, in bitter divorces.

Lovers or affairees (Doherty & Harris, 2017) are initially on their best behavior. And when they tell you how beautiful and brilliant you are, especially when you are also in the throes of passionate sex, it will be hard to think and see clearly. But there is a high probability that these lovers will prove to be just like the person you are trying to escape.

John claimed that his wife Charlotte was a demanding narcissist who only cared about getting her needs met. He said that she rarely showed affection to him or their children and never initiated sex. To get some much-needed attention, John began an affair with a single woman, Denise, who at the time seemed to be just what John needed: a soft, attentive, affectionate, and sensual woman. But following his divorce, John was shocked to discover that Denise proved just as narcissistic as his first wife. She demanded that he fight to reduce his alimony and child support so that she could afford a better lifestyle and had little to no empathy for his children, who grew to hate her. When not pleased, Denise would respond by withholding sex and soon began her own affair.

As you will see in Section III, Clinical Treatment of Unmet Expectations, for couples to change at a deep level, each partner must examine their respective families of origin, identify their shared internal master conflict, and differentiate enough to allow for integration of both sides of the conflict. This process will, in turn, reduce their symptoms.

References

Betchen, S. (2010). *Magnetic partners: Discover how the hidden conflict that once attracted you to each other is now driving you apart.* Free Press.

Betchen, S. (2022). *Couples in conflict: Clinical techniques for navigating sexual and relationship control struggles.* Routledge.

Betchen, S., & Davidson, H. L. (2018). *Master conflict therapy: A new model for practicing couples and sex therapy.* Routledge.

Doherty, W., & Harris, S. (2017). *Helping couples on the brink of divorce.* American Psychological Association.

World Population Review. (2022). Divorce data by state 2022. Retrieved from https://worldpopulationreview.com/staterankings/divorce-rate-by-state

4   Sociocultural Influences

Society

Talcott Parsons (1937/1968) viewed society as a system with four basic functions: adaptation, goal attainment, integration, and pattern maintenance. MacIver and Page (1949) defined society as an ever-changing, complex "system of usages and procedures, of authority and mutual aid, of many groupings and divisions, of controls of human behavior and of liberties" (p. 5). Durkheim (1973) believed that society held enormous influence over its individual members, and that in society people's norms, beliefs, and values make up a collective consciousness. He said of society:

> It requires that, forgetful of our own interests, we make ourselves its servitors, and it submits us to every sort of inconvenience, privation, and sacrifice, without which social life would be impossible. It is because of this that at every instant we are obliged to submit ourselves to rules of conduct and of thought which we have neither made nor desired, and which are sometimes even contrary to our most fundamental inclinations and instincts.
>
> (p. 169)

Given regional and relational proximity, and shared goals, it should come as no surprise that the expectations of a people are influenced by the society, or the philosophy of the society they are raised in and continue to live in. Communist societies expect their people to work for the benefit of the community, the political party, and the country. Personal interests should never be placed above these. In an industrialized, capitalistic society such as the United States, emphasis is placed on individual achievement, private ownership, and financial independence. Competition and personal success are of immense importance.

On the micro level, the expectations valued by a society inevitably impact its couples and can contribute to internalized conflicts. For example, two of the most common symptoms presented by couples, especially in capitalistic societies, are in the context of conflicts with money, and the balancing of work and family. In the following two sections notice that many of the examples, although they are recent, are still reflective of our society's traditional values in these two areas.

DOI: 10.4324/9781003359470-5

Money/Finances

According to Atwood (2012) and Shapiro (2007), money impacts the interactions in committed relationships. In the context of money, I am most often presented with three situations. The first is when one partner (usually the male in a hetero-sexual couple) is: 1) unemployed for too long a time through no fault of his own; 2) unemployed yet not actively looking for work; or 3) unable to earn enough to support his family. Sometimes this partner is working but spending more than he makes on things that his female counterpart considers non-essential such as a motorcycle or boat. The female partner might prefer that the couple instead pay for a new roof.

Whatever the specific situation, however, the female partner expects her mate to do his part and when he falls short, there is potential for trouble. In recent years I have had several cases in which the woman refuses to work even though the couple is experiencing financial problems and even though the man expects her to help. In such cases the woman might be hanging onto traditional values.

In a second example, the female complains that the male partner is withholding money from her or controlling the couple's finances – another holdover from traditional values. This is in sync with the most common complaint that men register: that women spend too much money, whether for good (e.g., to help family members or friends in need) or bad reasons (e.g., to spoil the children). In an extreme case, a husband confessed that he destroyed his wife's credit cards to curb her spending.

And in a third example, one or both partners may hide money, or they may spend it without the other knowing. Garbinsky et al. (2020) referred to this as "financial infidelity." They specifically defined the concept as: "engaging in any financial behavior expected to be disapproved of by one's romantic partner and intentionally failing to disclose this behavior to them" (p. 1). The authors even developed the Financial Infidelity Scale (FI-scale) to measure proneness for financial infidelity. This dynamic will be especially problematic if one partner is a "sharer" or "team player" and the other is not.

If partners have their respective conflicts with finances under control, it will be easy for them to work together to alleviate them. Specifically, there might be more empathy for the partner who is jobless, or the jobless partner will try harder to find a job. The controlling partner may become more judicious about how money is spent, or the couple can develop a budget or agree on how to spend their money; they may even agree to greater financial transparency.

If, however, the couple's shared conflict is unbalanced, financial symptoms will appear. For example, if a frugal partner expects her mate to save money but because of her own conflict unconsciously partners up with a spendthrift who resists control, lacks discipline, and has a pattern of financial irresponsibility, neither will have their expectations fulfilled. The frugal partner might expect the spendthrift to curb his ways. In response, the free spender might rebel and expect her to leave him to his own devices. Neither will have their financial expectations met.

A second example of this type of conflict is indicated if a partner of little means has risen beyond his/her circumstances and is in conflict about relying on others to offer a hand financially. While the struggle is painful, the satisfaction of succeeding on one's own is equally important. If the self-sufficient partner chooses someone from a wealthy, intrusive family who expects consistent family aid, the couple must maintain a fragile balance. The partner from the poor background will expect the other partner to work hard to build their own separate empire while the partner with the wealthy background expects family aid without strain.

A third example: a nonworking partner marries, has several children, and expects to stay home and care for them. The working partner, however, decides unilaterally to stop working. Rather than take a job, the nonworking partner responds to this by refusing to get a job and the couple fight over whose responsibility it is to support the family. The nonworking partner expects to be taken care of but unconsciously marries an angry individual who rebels or tends to be paralyzed by depression when times get tough. When trouble ensues, however, the beleaguered working partner then expects the nonworking partner to take on financial responsibility. In fact, the working partner insists upon it.

Work vs. Domestic/Family Obligations

Bruk (2019) warned: "The division of housework is one of the main sources of tension between cohabitating couples, one that even comes up as a reason for divorce" (p. 1). In the context of balancing work and family, typically, one partner (usually the female) might complain that her male counterpart is paying far too much attention to his career (e.g., seeking promotions, and making money) rather than spending time with the family and doing his share of the domestic chores. The males in these cases claim that their wives expect too much – that it is hard for them to earn the money they make and keep up with familial duties simultaneously. I usually hear something like: "You want me to spend less time at work, but you don't seem to mind driving a Mercedes Benz."

If each partner's conflict with expectations is balanced, they can usually negotiate a compromise between work and family life. But if they are unbalanced, a chronic control struggle can develop in this context that can leave both partners with unmet needs. The following are examples of unbalanced conflicts in the context of unmet expectations.

If one partner is overworking and expecting his partner to be supportive in his endeavors, he might ironically put the very thing he has worked so hard for – to create a kingdom for he and his family – at risk if his marriage fails. The conflict frequently manifests when a workaholic marries someone whose main purpose is to create a close-knit family. She expects her husband to be an integral part of the family but his goal, which has been the same from the very beginning of their relationship, is to work. He claims that he works to support the family. This is partially true, but he also works because it offers him self-esteem and self-worth, buys him a certain amount of distance from his partner and family, and because he likes to work.

A second example is of the young man who marries and has children yet insists on living like an unmarried person. He hangs out with his friends, extends his athletic career, and spends several hours at the bars and clubs of his early youth. I have seen men like this who participate in team sports all year round, well into their forties and fifties, or until they rupture an Achilles tendon. This individual expects to be taken care of or left alone to have fun. One young man said to his wife: "I am the head of the household. Back off and stop trying to tell me what to do." The wife responded with: "Well, if you want to be the man, act like one."

If this man was not in conflict with his expectations, he would have married a woman who was not in conflict with enabling his extended childhood. Instead, he married a serious, caretaking mother-figure whose conflict was made evident by her disdain for being taken advantage of. Women like this often say to me: "I have three children I do not want another." If the therapist digs deep enough, most of these men will admit what they are doing is wrong and they need to step up and help their counterparts. This is especially true of those with children.

A third example, and the closest representative of traditional values is that of a man who has rigid gender roles. That is, he thinks that women should take responsibility for "inside the home" (e.g., cooking, cleaning) and men should take care of "outside the home" (e.g., cutting grass, keeping the cars running). When two partners are not in conflict, all goes well, and each partner fulfills their roles to keep the family functioning. When in conflict, however. a man like this may partner up with a woman who sees these roles from a more egalitarian perspective. That is, whatever needs tending to, whoever is freed up, should take care of it. This man claims to want a traditional wife but unconsciously chooses a feminist. He likes her feistiness but expects her to play a more traditional role. The woman in conflict may be attracted to a man's toughness and initially forget she is opposed to rigid gender roles. She expects a man to take care of her when she decides it is necessary, but otherwise she wants to be his equal.

Changes in Society

The previous examples reflected the traditional values of our society. But while it usually takes generations, societies can change and with it, the expectations of its people. For example, following the Civil Rights Movement of the 1960s, women have achieved more equality with men. According to the Pew Research Center, women are more educated than ever, and they outnumber men in college (Parker, 2021). Bryant (2022) found that women aged 25 years and older are more likely to hold a four-year degree than men. This will eventually translate to more women in graduate and professional schools than men. Women now make up approximately 47% of the workforce which is up 30% from 1950, and a growing number are breadwinners in their families (Geiger & Parker, 2018).

New research has even indicated that young women (i.e., under age 30) are out-earning young men in many U.S. cities (Fry, 2022).

There is still, however, an overall gender pay gap favoring men in the work world. According to the Harvard Business Review, as of 2022 women earned 17% less than men on average. Controlling for lower-paying occupations, gender bias, and a reluctance to pursue higher pay, it was found that outside or domestic obligations still led to unpredictable schedules and in turn, lower pay for women (Bolotnyy & Emanual, 2022).

There is no denying that women are no longer as dependent on men as they once were and are even marrying less frequently. Traditionally most women longed for marriage – for many it was their chief goal – now many feel it is better to stay single and independent rather than to subjugate themselves in a relationship. According to the U.S. Census Bureau over the last 10 years the marriage rate has decreased. In 2019 there were 16.5 new marriages per every 1,000 women aged 15 and over in the U.S., down from 17.6 in 2009 (Anderson & Scherer, 2020).

On the home front, men are participating more in domestic chores such as cooking and grocery shopping, but women still take on the bulk of domestic responsibilities (Schaeffer, 2019). These findings have even held up during the pandemic. In one large study, 59% of the women claimed they did more of the housework than their male partners, while only 6% said that their partner did more (Barroso, 2021). Now that women work more and earn more, have high stress jobs, and lead companies, they take offense when they must do the bulk of the childcare and housework; this is especially true if their male counterparts are not employed. It is also appalling to many women when men argue that because they earn more, they should do less at home and with the children. But I have heard men offer this same defense in households in which women are clearly the primary breadwinners.

In households free of internal conflict with expectations, couples can more easily accept societal changes and their impact on gender roles. But those in conflict can just as easily produce relationship symptoms. Women, for example, might want equality but experience guilt when not taking sole responsibility for the jobs they were traditionally assigned by society. Even millennial women report that they feel guilty when earning more than their male counterparts (Ford, 2017). I have treated women who sabotage their own success so as not to intimidate or scare off the men in their lives. Although a woman I treated was clearly far more educated than her husband and made twice his salary, she spent the entire session telling him how much smarter he was than her.

Men in conflict, however, may want to spend more time at home but feel they might be less competitive in the work world and fail to fulfill the traditional masculine role traditionally assigned to them. Syrda (2019) found that male stress levels rise if their female counterparts earn 40% of the household income. Males still prefer to be breadwinners, in part, to preserve their masculine ideal. Even gay men have been known to fight over breadwinner status (Howard, 2016). The following case would have once been considered an outlier but today it is common:

Ellen was the Senior Vice President of a large company. She made a very lucrative living and was the breadwinner in a family of five. Ellen admitted that she liked to be in charge just as her mother was in her family of origin. But she simultaneously claimed she did not want to emasculate a man and so along with her demanding job she took on the bulk of the housework and childrearing.

Ellen's husband Bart, an exceptionally talented sculptor, barely made a living, nor did he try. You might think that Ellen would be the initiator of treatment, but it was Bart who insisted on couples therapy under the guise that Ellen was asexual.

Ellen disagreed with her husband's diagnosis as the couple were having quality sex twice per week. But Bart did not think that was enough. He wanted sex several times a week even though Ellen was simply too busy and exhausted to accommodate him.

It was clear in treatment that Bart was not interested in working too hard at anything and expected to be taken care of by Ellen. Ellen, in conflict about being the boss of her husband, could not set any limits with him. She did not expect him to earn a living or take on more of the household responsibilities.

It was only when Bart began to focus on his conflict about what he expected of himself as a married man and father that he began to deal with his own shortcomings and to stop using sex as a defense against his conflict.

Culture

Anthropologist Edward Burnett Tylor (1873/2016) defined culture as: "Culture or Civilization, taken in its wide ethnographic sense, is that complex whole which includes knowledge, belief, art, morals, law, custom, and any other capabilities and habits acquired by man as a member of society" (p. 1). Malinowski (2013) pointed out: "Each culture owes its completeness and self-sufficiency to the fact that it satisfies the whole range of basic, instrumental and integrative needs" (p. 40). In connecting it more closely to human behavior, Marsella and Yamada (2010) wrote:

Culture is shared learned behavior and meanings that are socially transmitted for purposes of adjustment and adaptation. Culture is represented externally in artifacts (e.g., food, clothing, music), roles (e.g., the social formation), and institutions (e.g., family, government). It is represented internally (e.g., cognitively, emotionally) by values, attitudes, beliefs, epistemologies, cosmologies, consciousness patterns, and notions of personhood. Culture is coded in verbal imagistically, proprioceptively, viscerally, and emotionally, resulting in different experiential structures and processes.

(p. 105)

Given these definitions it is no wonder why people from diverse cultures see life from different perspectives and behave in accordance with their views. The United States prides itself on being a multicultural nation. According to an analysis of data from the U.S. Bureau of the Census, as of 2022 there were 46.6 million immigrants in America (Camarota & Zeigler, 2022). This represents 14.2% of the total population, the highest in over one hundred years. The authors predict that if current trends continue, the immigrant share is likely to surpass the all-time highs recorded in 1890 (14.6%) and in 1910 (14.7%) in the next few years.

With so many foreign-born people of diverse cultures coming together in American society, and with their own distinct ways passed onto them through their various cultures, it is vital for therapists to understand and to respect their varied beliefs, customs, morals, and values. Kreuz and Roberts (2017) contended that the communicational styles of couples from diverse cultures, both verbal and nonverbal, are also vital in better understanding relational dynamics.

It is also important to consider that many of these attitudes and beliefs will be passed on to their American-born children in subsequent generations. This is, in part, why most psychotherapists need to work hard to embrace and adapt to these changes by familiarizing themselves with the ways of others. According to Lee and Park (2013), the values in therapy often come into direct conflict with the values of a multicultural population. And several scholars claim that it is not difficult for the therapist to miss cultural-related cues and values (Lee, 2015; Lee & Bhuyan, 2013; Lee & Horvath, 2013, 2014).

Bhugra and De Silva (2000) contended that cultural differences are especially challenging in couple therapy because of the many ways they can manifest. It is agreed upon by many therapists that understanding the role of factors such as culture is necessary for the couples therapist to join with and assess couples (Falconier et al., 2016; Falicov, 2014; Jordan & Carlson, 2013; Karis & Killian, 2009; Kelly, 2017; Rastogi & Thomas, 2009; Zaker & Boostanipoor, 2016). Because all couples have both expectations and conflicts, this model is applicable to couples of all cultural backgrounds. The following are some examples of couples where their conflict with expectations was influenced by their cultural backgrounds:

American-Born Greek Man and American-Born Greek Woman

While it is common in our society for women to want children, this is especially true in cultures that place even more emphasis on creating a family, such as Mediterranean cultures. Lydia, a second-generation Greek American woman I was treating, claimed that her father, a native Greek man was so controlling of her and that she would never again give up that kind of control to anyone, including a future spouse. She realized that it was normal for the Greek patriarchal culture, but rather than obey this tradition she decided to rebel. Instead of marrying and having children, she chose to pursue higher education and career success. While her family was proud of Lydia's achievements, they still considered them secondary to marrying and having children. And they often expressed disappointment in Lydia for not following their cultural traditions.

While most of her life consisted of battles with her father, as she aged Lydia began to miss being in a long-term relationship and having children. But every time she entered a relationship, she soon became embroiled in a control struggle with whoever she happened to be dating. The fights were mostly over her lack of commitment, distancing, and her extreme sensitivity to even the most constructive criticism. It was evident when Lydia presented for couples therapy that she expected her boyfriend, Nico at that time, also an American-born Greek, to put up with her behavior regardless of his feelings or desires. But being raised in a patriarchal system Nico refused to comply.

Evason's (2019) findings support the dynamics of Lydia's case. The author contended that Greek society has been traditionally male dominated, that the Greek family is considered "the most important foundation of their society, providing emotional and economic support to the individual" (p. 1). Having a son to continue the family name is highly valued. Evason also claimed that the Greek population has been on the decline; this is a piece of information that Lydia's father used on Lydia to convince her to have a child. While this did not work, it did contribute to Lydia's conflict.

Lydia's conflict with expectations revealed that while she expected men to meet her needs unconditionally, she was simultaneously sabotaging her chances of this. The older she got the harder her unresolved conflict was to address, in part because her childbearing years had passed.

American-Born Italian Man and American-Born Italian Woman

A patriarchal culture demands certain expectations of men. For example, I treated an Italian man, Anthony, who was a second-generation Italian American. Anthony had slept with many women before and after he married. He saw no harm or sin in infidelity. However, after he requested a trial separation to be with one of his many lovers, his wife, Donna, thinking her marriage was over, decided to begin dating.

Finding out that his wife was dating, however, infuriated Anthony and he immediately countered by insisting that the couple resume their marriage. While Donna cautiously agreed, Anthony proved to be so irate that she had dated (even though she had yet to sleep with anyone) he could not refrain from constant name calling and shaming her. He insisted, for example, that Donna was a disloyal "slut."

When I questioned Anthony's double standard, he was surprised to find that, as a man, I did not side with him on this issue. He had no real explanation for his attitude other than it was a normal one for him to have. In his world, the husband should expect his wife to allow him to do whatever he wants and yet remain faithful to him. Anthony was so entrenched in this culturally influenced belief, passed down from his father and grandfather, that it made it almost impossible for him to forgive his wife.

This attitude in Italian men is supported by numerous studies. For example, a large survey conducted by the French Institute of Public Opinion and Gleeden (a French dating site for people looking to have affairs) found that 55% of Italian men – tied with French men for the highest rates in Europe – admitted to cheating on their spouses. And of all European men, only 26% of Italian men were regretful – the lowest number (Huffpost, 2014). According to data from the Pew Research Center only 64% of Italians found adultery unacceptable (Wike, 2014).

In a moment of insight Donna told Anthony that his Italian sense of masculinity would not let him forgive her. She added even though Anthony left her, and that she had never cheated on him, she had still broken a sacred cultural taboo passed down to him by his dictatorial Sicilian born father, and older brothers. Nevertheless, even her American Italian parents expected her to put up with Anthony's infidelities.

American-Born WASP Woman and Arab-born Man (Jordanian)

Amir was born and raised in Jordan. He sometimes lived in other parts of the Middle East but never outside of it until he decided to come to the United States to seek his fortune. During that time, Amir met Sally, a nice Christian woman with Mayflower roots, and the two initially formed what they thought was a passionate bond of complementary opposites. Sally was quiet, dignified, and self-contained while Amir was charismatic, friendly, and sure of himself. Amir could also be hot-tempered if he felt disrespected.

The couple presented for treatment because Sally was threatening divorce. She claimed that Amir was controlling and jealous. She also said that she felt "trapped" as if there was a "noose tightening around her neck." Even when Amir spoke to her, he constantly touched her, and she felt as if her personal space was being invaded. She summed up Amir's communication style as "nose to nose."

Sally was first attracted to Amir's attention to her, and she expected this to continue but in a less intense manner. Simply put, she loved having most of her needs met but expected Amir to back off if she asked him to. Instead, he would close the space between them even more.

Amir was upset by Sally's analysis of their relationship. He claimed that he deeply loved Sally and that he was not trying to trap her. He said that he enjoyed being with his wife all the time and that he could not understand why she needed space from him. He said where he came from, it was a sign of love to want to spend as much time with your wife as possible, and that his jealousy was only meant to protect their relationship from intruders. At one point he questioned: "What is wrong with loving your wife so much?"

Amir sensed that Sally needed someone to show a lot of interest in her given she came from an emotionally disengaged family. He expected her to respond positively to his constant attention and to appreciate and understand the level of intensity he brought to a relationship. He claimed to be shocked by her need for distance and especially that she was considering ending their marriage. He added that family was everything, and that he did not believe in divorce. While Amir wanted to be married to an independent, professional American woman who could help him to succeed, he also expected her to be more subservient. He certainly did not plan to pay for this by having a distant wife.

Anthropologist Edward T. Hall (1990a) wrote:

> People have developed their territoriality to an almost unbelievable extent. Yet we treat space as we treat sex. It is there but we don't talk about it. And if we do, we certainly are not expected to get technical or serious about it.
>
> (p. 159)

Hall coined the term *proxemics* to represent "the interrelated observations and theories of man's use of space as a specialized elaboration of culture" (1990b, p.1). In interviewing many people from across the globe, he examined various forms of distance such as intimate, personal, social, and public distance. In tune with Amir's perspective, Hall found that Arabs required far less intimate and personal distance when communicating than would an American like Sally. In fact, Hall found that to some Arabs too much space was arrogant or insulting. Therefore, it would make perfect sense to him given each partner's cultural background that Amir would reflexively close the distance between he and Sally, and for Sally to feel controlled, intimidated or threatened by this proximity. Kreuz and Roberts (2017) support the concept that people of distinct cultures are comfortable with varying degrees of interpersonal space.

American-Born Jewish Woman and Israeli-Born Man

I have also seen many Jewish-American women who felt pressured to marry within their faith. To appease their parents most conform but the tragedy is that many do so at the cost of "love." The professions are highly valued in Jewish culture and many young women were trained from an early age that it is beneficial to marry a professional man. While this is not a terrible thing in of itself, in my experience some comply regardless of how they feel about the man. Some of these women have broken up with men who did not fit expectations only to marry someone they had little passion for. This lack of love and sometimes even physical attraction seem to be reasons some of these individuals focus too heavily on their children.

Under pressure to marry a Jewish man, I have treated numerous couples in which a Jewish-American women decided to take things to the next level and marry an Israeli man. While this might sit well in the Jewish-American community, there can be a significant difference between the Israeli view of life and the suburban American Jewish way of life.

Ari, an Israeli man felt the need to remind his wife, Carole, that vacuuming the living room would not kill her. He then went on to say that in Israel, his mother did the bulk of the housework and never complained. He added that he expected her to do the same. He called them "real women." Ari was also quick to point out that overall, his family does a lot more for them than his in-laws do. Ari expected his Jewish in-laws to be at least as financially supportive as his parents were. And last, Ari was especially upset with what he saw as his wife's withholding of sex from him. He believed that it was a wife's duty to have sex with her husband when he wanted it, and that he was perplexed because he thought American women were sexually liberated.

Carole's response was to tell Ari what he already knew – that her mother did little housework because her family always had a house cleaner. She then cursed at him and told him that it was his job to make enough money to hire a house cleaning service. She also said it was not her parents' responsibility to support them on a continuous basis. Carole reminded Ari that given her father helped him to start a business in the United States, he could afford a house cleaner. This was Carole's way of telling Ari that she fulfilled his major expectation: to help him live the American Dream, but that he had to accept some limitations. She also told him that if he didn't stop trying to make her into an Israeli woman, he would never get sex from her again.

Ari's conflict dictated that he would pursue the American dream and expect help from a family that would make it come true. But he also expected his wife to act and perform like he thought an American-Jewish woman should. Carole's conflict dictated that she would expect to please her parents and her local community by marrying a man within her faith. But she also expected to be treated equally or better.

The dynamics of this case was supported by The Jewish News of Northern California (1997) which claimed that when Jewish women marry Israeli men, they soon find the close ties the Israelis have with their families and especially their mothers, are factors for life. According to data from the Pew Research Center, 73% of Israelis say that being connected to one's family is central to Jewish identity. And while this can be perceived initially as supportive by American women, with time it can be felt as intrusive (Sahgal & Cooperman, 2016). This is not so true in American families where they expect their children to be more independent after being launched.

Also, according to an article entitled: *We need to talk about how Israeli men treat American women*, Singer (2018) confirmed that Israeli men see American Jewish women as sexually promiscuous. The author also pointed out that Israeli men see these women as sexual prizes or possessions. Brodie (2019) validated this claim by suggesting that misogyny is deep-rooted in the Israeli male.

American-born Man and Columbian-Born Woman

Valentina was born and raised in Columbia. She left in part because of the violence she had experienced both in the crime-ridden streets and at the hands of her father and subsequent boyfriends. She eventually found a home in South Carolina and married an older man, Donald, hoping for a better life in which she was treated as an equal.

Donald, an attorney from a prominent WASP background, was a staid, stoic individual who claimed that his family was drama-free but lacking in adventure and spontaneity. But when he introduced this South American beauty to family members, they were not so welcoming. They saw Valentina as a "gold digger," and were dismissive of her. Valentina was a street-smart person and noticed even the most subtle of their insults. But instead of gently challenging what she believed were jealous, less attractive women, she would lose her temper and confront those she believed offended her. Donald was appalled by this behavior and often failed to support her.

Valentina viewed America as a less patriarchal system than Columbia, thus she expected to be treated as an equal by her husband. And because she was also from a family-oriented culture she expected that all family members would welcome her with open arms and that she could feel safe and secure. But when she got none of this she was shattered. Donald, on the other hand, expected that because Valentina was younger, and came from a poorer background and a patriarchal country, she would be thankful for what he could provide for her. He also expected little resistance from her and that he would be the boss. Valentina said that he expected a pretty little doll who would look good on his arm and travel with him rather than a woman with her own ideas.

Like Valentina, research has indicated that many Columbian women have left their country in part because of social violence and political upheaval (Madrigal, 2013). They also experience violence in their own homes at the hands of men. This is in part why many Columbian women who have experienced this violence prefer less machismo partners (Borras-Guevara, Batres, & Perrett, 2019). Columbian men also are said to treat Columbian women like servants and these women yearn for caring and respect (European Business Review, 2022).

Columbian women are typically considered passionate, family-oriented, and intensely loyal to their partners. But with this also comes a fiery side and arguments can seem much more serious to their foreign partners than the Columbian women would perceive it (Expatgroup.co, 2021; Gonzalez, 2020). What Valentina saw as a passionate discussion, Donald saw as destructive conflict, and so did his family who began to distance themselves from the couple. Llerena-Quinn and Bacigalupe (2009) described this dynamic in the case of the Latino woman Nora and her American husband Richard:

> Richard, from a WASP background, felt overwhelmed with all the display of emotion, which looked to him like a "fight." He could not understand how

Nora's family could intensely disagree, raise their voices, and then go onto the next thing as if nothing had happened. He, instead, like his family, was reserved and polite, never expressing strong opinions, much less criticism.

(p. 182)

Israeli-Born Man and Israeli-Born Woman

People from the same cultures have an edge when it comes to knowing what to expect from each other. But getting it can be a different story. Aviva was born and raised in Israel and served in the Israeli army. She was assertive and would never fail to tell you what was on her mind. You didn't need to guess what Aviva was thinking even if you were a friend, but especially if you were her husband.

Aviva married her husband Uri in Israel and came to America to start a business and live a better life. In treatment, Aviva was chiefly upset with Uri because she felt he still acted like a child and took little responsibility at home or with the children. It seemed as if she was always scolding him for something. Uri was a good provider, but he was like a big kid. But rather than distance from Aviva, he would take on her every challenge and argue with her whether he was right or wrong.

Aviva was a shrewd businessperson who helped Uri build his business, but he always fought her input even if it meant he would make some serious financial mistakes. Aviva was more cautious and calculating and Uri would impulsively jump into action without thinking of the potential consequences. Aviva insisted that Uri attend the couples therapy with her. She revealed that while most Israeli men were babied by their mothers, she thought Uri was different. She expected Uri to act more like a man than a little boy. She said she was tired of being a mother to him. She especially claimed that she hated having to nag Uri. She found it embarrassing and degrading to both. Uri admitted that Israeli women are not generally passive, and they usually have a big say in family life. But he acted as if he expected Aviva to baby him as his mother did and let him do whatever he wanted to do. Aviva refused to do so.

Studies suggest that Israeli women still face sexism in Israel (Cohen-Almagor & Maroshek-Klarman, 2022) although they have made some gains in matters not related to religious values and norms. They are also known for speaking their minds, as Aviva did.

While Israeli couples tend to fight often, ironically this does necessarily interfere with their sex lives, and there is rarely talk of divorce. Winkler and Doherty (1983) found that Israeli couples may fight a lot, but this does not impact their marital satisfaction as it does in American couples. Aviva and Uri fought frequently but this did not seem to interfere with their affection for one another, and there was no indication that their problems would ever lead to an end to the relationship. Israel is also a "child-centered" society (Marciano, 2019) that promotes closeness to one's parents and extended family well into adulthood (Bar-Tur et al., 2018). There is, however, nothing significant in the literature to back up Aviva's claim that Israeli mothers spoil their sons.

Arab-born Man and Arab-Born Woman (Lebanese)

Samir and his wife Fatima were born and raised in Lebanon and only recently came to the United States so that Fatima could complete her graduate studies. Samir was in the computer business in Lebanon, so it was easy for him to move it to the United States.

Samir reluctantly came to therapy even though he agreed with Fatima that their marriage was suffering from endless arguments. Samir was a traditional man and he believed that his wife was too domineering. He expected to always have the last word in his marriage and believed that it was his right to have it given he was the man of the family. If it were up to him, he would not have sought treatment. He was embarrassed by this need and had a challenging time showing his vulnerable side.

Fatima countered that she did not want to emasculate Samir, and certainly did not want to dominate him. She even admitted that a passive man would not have attracted her. But she did add that she was a highly educated woman, valued having an opinion, and that she expected more respect from her husband. When they first met, Fatima said that Samir showed her a gentle, liberal, and relaxed style, but when they married, he became more patriarchal. Samir claimed that he does respect Fatima but that she is too bossy and has an opinion on everything. He added that when dating, Fatima showed him a more passive side even though he knew she could be outspoken at times. He expected a more passive wife.

This dynamic is not surprising given that the literature on Lebanese couples suggests that despite their many attributes such as loyalty and family-orientation, Lebanese men have a challenging time being vulnerable, as did Samir. According to Semaan (2016), Lebanese men have been raised by their mothers to be tough and in fact could be scolded if they cried. This in part accounts for their macho attitudes that still permeate Lebanese culture which many Lebanese women have been fighting.

In an interview for the United Nations (2022) article entitled *The Fight for Gender Equality in Lebanon*, Claudia Aoun, President of the National Commission for Lebanese Women stated:

> Women are singly not recognized as citizens the way men are. We have had some advances on women's equality but the citizenship issue remains a taboo. This can be traced in part to the confessional system and political parties at a stalemate: what one group considers discrimination; another sees as culture.
>
> (p.1)

Asian-Born Man and Asian-Born Woman (Indian)

Darsh and his wife Prisha, were both born and raised in India. After their marriage was arranged both decided to come to the United States to complete their masters' degrees in computer science and engineering respectfully. The couple presented for couple's work primarily because Darsh felt that his wife gave up most of their country's customs soon after she arrived in America, and that both sets of parents were upset by this. They were especially worried that their customs would not be passed on to their grandchildren. This did not concern Prisha. In fact, she said that did not want her daughter to be raised in a system that oppresses women. Prisha wanted to be more liberated, and this was one of the main reasons for coming to America.

Prisha expected Darsh to respect her wishes since she said that he always seemed to respect women's rights compared to the men she knew in India. She also expected him to support her in battling with the parents even though she did not necessarily want to alienate them. Darsh insisted that he was more liberal than his friends, but that Prisha's rebelliousness was irritating his parents and in turn they were putting pressure on him to get Prisha to conform. Her parents seemed to have given up fighting her. Darsh knew that Prisha wanted a say in their marriage and he was prepared for this. But he was not prepared to give up his culture and his parents' approval for her. He did not expect her to put her values ahead of him, their cultural heritage, their family, and their marriage.

According to Chadda and Deb (2013), "Indian society is collectivist and promotes social cohesion and interdependence" (p. S299). Thus, it would make sense that Indian parents and grandparents have a great deal of influence on their children well into adulthood. And because Indian culture is hierarchal and patriarchal, Indian men are seen as the primary decisionmakers. This is supported by data from the Pew Research Center which indicates that most Indians (67%) still believe that Indian women should obey their husbands. Indian women are only slightly less likely to feel the same way (61%). And four in ten Indian people believe that traditional gender roles are best (Evans et al., 2022). Given this data it was clear to see why Prisha's independent, feminist perspective was not well-received, especially by the elders of her family, and why her husband was viewed by them as weak.

Irish-Born Woman and Egyptian-Born Man

It is usually even more complicated for a therapist to treat a couple consisting of two partners each from foreign and contrasting cultures. Not only would there then be two cultures to consider but the therapist might add a third – his or hers. Fiona was born and raised in Belfast, Ireland and her husband Ahmed was born and raised in Egypt. Both met while working abroad and although they maintained a long-distance relationship for three years, they finally came together in the United States.

It was Fiona's idea to seek therapy because she said she was at her wits end with Ahmed and she was ready to divorce. Fiona claimed that her husband acted as if he was always right, and that he believed that he should be able to use their money as he pleased. Ahmed countered that family in his culture was most important and that helping his relatives, especially his parents, took priority over his personal financial concerns. Fiona said that she understood this but that they were on the verge of bankruptcy because Ahmed was constantly throwing money at his family. She even claimed that he bought two cars for them without consulting her.

Ahmed went as far as to say his wife was being disrespectful to him because he was the man and should be able to make these decisions without her sanctioning. This would provoke Fiona, who had quite a temper, and she would curse at Ahmed. Fiona expected to have a close family, but she did not expect that it would be as close as it is. Ahmed thought that Fiona wanted a close family but did not expect her to try and dictate the parameters. He also unconsciously underestimated Fiona's independent streak and toughness. He saw this as a threat to his masculinity. Fiona unconsciously underestimated Ahmed's patriarchal attitudes and his intense loyalty to his Egyptian family.

According to Betts (2022), modern Egypt is still collectivist, and the family is of the utmost importance. Children are considered a blessing, and obligations to parents and extended family are expected to be fulfilled until they die; sons, as Ahmed demonstrated, are especially tasked with this cultural obligation (Okasha et al., 2012).

Egyptian men are also considered the heads of their households and the prime decision makers in their families. This supports their masculine identity and sometimes machismo behavior (Abdelmoez, 2018). Ahmed took the role as decision maker in his marriage, and in part this explains why he saw nothing wrong with not telling his wife about sending money to his family in Egypt. This, however, was not Fiona's Irish experience, and so she took his behavior as a controlling betrayal.

Religion

Studies have shown that religiosity, especially shared religious practice, and values are closely related to marital satisfaction in both Western and other cultures (Aman et al., 2019; David & Stafford, 2015; Sauerheber et al., 2020). However, religion and religious differences can also serve as the context for conflicts with expectations in couples. The following examples depict this:

Christian Man and Christian Woman (Methodist)

Anytime there are institutions involved, complying with the norm is encouraged and expected. According to Dee (2015), there are several reasons why Christians marry Christians: 1) it is what the Bible says to do; 2) because they view the world the same; 4) because they view themselves as the same; 5) because both partners view marriage the same; and 6) because they answer to the same authority. While Dee makes a case against interfaith marriage, other factors can be at play that complicate matters. The following description of a case will illustrate this:

A young woman raised in a strong Christian environment, Sara, was urged to marry into her faith. As regular church goers, her family's social life revolved around the church. When old enough, Sara acquiesced and married a good Christian man, William, whom she met at her church. William met every requirement on Sara's check list: He was a good Christian, handsome, a good provider, and seemed likely to make a good father and loyal husband. And he was all of these. Unfortunately, however, Sara never considered whether she was physically attracted to him. In fact, she said that attraction and passion were not on her check list.

William was a genuinely nice man, but Sara was not in the least attracted to him. Even more painful was the fact that because this woman's religion and family frowned upon divorce, she felt trapped in her situation. William was disappointed and disturbed to discover that his wife no longer wanted him, yet he still preferred to stay with her. Both partners were in conflict. Sara wanted to move on but knew she was expected to live with her choice. William expected his wife to love him or at least to stay in a loveless relationship, but she was having difficulty doing this.

Jewish Man and Christian Woman (Lutheran)

Intermarriage is a complicated process but still on the rise. According to a study conducted by the Pew Research Center (2021), 42% of currently married Jewish respondents said they have a non-Jewish spouse. And of those who have gotten married since 2010, 61% are intermarried. But despite its increasing commonality, the interfaith marriage between a Christian and a Jew often merits ongoing negotiation, and a compromise of goals, values, and sometimes lifestyle. According to the Jewish Women's Archive (2010), a Jew and a Christian have a 40% chance of divorce, while two Christians have a 20% chance.

Mark was a young Jewish man who fell in love with his high school sweetheart, Emma. Emma was Christian and of German heritage, of which she was quite proud. Emma's parents and extended family were upset when she brought Mark home to meet them and Mark's parents reacted to Emma in kind. Mark's mother made a negative comment about Emma's long blonde hair and blue eyes being too Aryan for her taste.

Considering themselves modern and free of prejudice they tried to fend off both sets of parents and maintain objectivity, but soon Emma decided that she wanted Mark to reduce the time he spent practicing his religion. For example, she no longer wanted either of them to attend Synagogue on the High Holidays. Emma considered this to be highlighting the differences between them and only making it harder for their families to accept them as a couple. Mark reacted strongly to this and expected Emma to allow him to at the very least pray in the holidays.

The couple sought treatment because they could not get out of this bind and Emma was threatening to end their relationship. Once in treatment both Emma and Mark realized that expecting each other to make these sacrifices was not going to work. And if they married and had children, they could not expect a compromise on how to raise them religiously. They were upset they didn't see this earlier, but their conflicts would not allow them to.

Race

The concept of race is fast being recognized as a significant factor that therapists are encouraged to consider in their practices. The therapist must be ready to treat all couples that are present for treatment and cultivate the empathy, knowledge, and skill to join with such couples for the good of the therapeutic process. Even though the distinctness of couples should be considered in therapy (Helm & Carlson, 2013), couples generally struggle with the same problems (Allen & Helm, 2013), and all have expectations. That is one major reason why this model is effective. The following examples illustrate how couples of different races are impacted by and struggle with unmet expectations:

Black Man and Black Woman

Keisha and Terrell were a young Black couple in their late 30s. Keisha had recently left Terrell because he was not helping her with the domestic chores and her three children from a prior marriage. Keisha said that when she first met Terrell he acted as if he were a responsible man. But soon she realized that Terrell was as much a child as her children, and she had had enough. She expected to be married to a "man."

Terrell was raised by a doting mother; his father had left home when he was an infant. When he first met Keisha, Terrell said she seemed as if she would be happy to take full control of their domestic responsibilities and he would only have to hold down a job. He expected her to be more like his mother. His unconscious allowed him to vastly underestimate Keisha's strength. Keisha underestimated Terrell's ability or desire to change into a more responsible adult. Unconsciously Terrell mated with another mother-figure and expected as much from her. Keisha got another child and a greater burden.

Black Man and White Woman

According to data from the Pew Research Center, one-in-ten newlyweds in the United States were married to a person of a different race or ethnicity in 2015, an increase from 3% in 1970. There is a total of 11 million intermarried people in the United States. There is also a significant reduction in non-Black people who oppose marrying a Black person down from 63% in 1990 to 14% in 2016. And newlywed Black men are twice as likely to intermarry as newlywed Black women, 24% compared to 12% (Bialik, 2017). Nevertheless, interracial couples must cope with negotiating gender roles, poor communication, differences with economic management, intimacy issues, managing societal disapproval, and, as in the case of Eric and Cynthia, managing the effects of racial privilege. Internal conflict only exacerbates these issues.

Eric and his young wife Cynthia dated for approximately one year and only recently married. They are yet to have children. Not being sure that Cynthia would date a Black man Eric was surprised when she said yes, especially because it was evident to him that she was from a much higher socioeconomic level. While all was fine for a time, Cynthia began to slowly complain that she did not like Rap Music, no longer would attend any concerts with Eric, and did not appreciate some of Eric's friends.

Cynthia expected that Eric would capitulate to her desires and, according to her, refine his tastes. Instead, Eric accused Cynthia of being racist and said that he expected much more from her. He told her that he did not like most of her "uppity white friends" who are spoiled and look down on him, but that he socialized with them for her sake. Both Eric and Cynthia's stances should not have come as a surprise because Eric's mother has been a long-time activist for Black equal rights and Cynthia's parents were of a country club set. Adding to the couple's shared conflict with expectations, neither set of parents were thrilled with the union but were at least respectful enough to let the young couple sort it out.

Asian Man and Asian Woman (Chinese)

While it is common for Chinese parents to "train" their children to achieve academically, it is not so common for anyone to see a Chinese family in overt distress (Chao, 1994; Fei-Yin Ng & Wei, 2020; Liu & Wang, 2015; Tanap, 2019). In fact, it is uncommon to see Chinese couples in therapy. According to Tanap (2019), the Chinese have been trained in their culture not to show weakness or vulnerability; they see it as a burden to express their emotions. Some Chinese may view complaining as a sign that they are ungrateful for all that they have. The following couple were in dire need of treatment but their shared conflict with expectations in conjunction with their cultural background made the process next to impossible.

Cheng and his wife Mei were a Chinese couple in their forties with three children of varying ages. While neither were happy about being in the couples therapy they were encouraged to go by their attorney because two of their children, who had their own therapists, had engaged in minor criminal activity. Their youngest child suffered from anxiety, and Mei was clearly depressed. While the couple had been married for many years and worked closely together in a family-owned business, Mei was gradually distancing from her husband and sinking into deeper depression.

The first problem that came up in treatment was scheduling – something the couple never could reconcile. Cheng claimed repeatedly that he could not afford to take time off from work and he expected that I and his wife would understand this. Because I knew that he was quite successful, I challenged Cheng's excuse but with no help from Mei. Mei just sat there with her head down looking sadder for the moment. Even when I warned Cheng that his marriage may be falling apart, he would not relent; he expected superhuman efforts from himself and all his family members.

We only managed two sessions before Cheng prematurely terminated and Mei dutifully followed him. While Cheng was a great provider, he was also a workaholic who expected perfection and utmost dedication to achieving it from himself, his wife, and his children. His main concern other than his work was making sure his children keep their grades up, but this wasn't happening either.

Cheng wanted respect from his wife and children, but he was working at cross-purposes because he could not understand that they had their limits. It was clear that as demanding as Cheng was, Mei was the opposite. As a passive and depressed woman, she hated what was happening to herself and her family and wanted badly to respect her husband, but she had little confidence in her ability to challenge his power. She expected that nothing could or would change.

Sex Orientation

I have not had enough experience with transgender couples to write with any authority about them. But I do have significant experience with gay couples who face many of the same problems all couples do but exacerbated by any discrimination they must endure (Connolly, 2012). This prejudice is said to be related to societal, biological, familial, and psychosocial factors (Dworkin & Pope, 2012), some of which have resulted in psychological, spiritual, and physical issues as well as work-related problems, and problems in their communities (Singh & Durso, 2017).

One of the most common issues that I see gay and lesbian couples struggling with, is when one or both partners are conflicted about being gay or homophobic. Homophobia is defined as an acceptance of society's antigay homophobic attitudes which can cause serious relationship problems and deter the coming out process (Frost & Meyer, 2010; Weber-Gilmore et al., 2014). The following two examples demonstrate what can happen when a couple have conflicted expectations in the context of homophobia.

Gay Male Couple

Michael was a handsome gay man with an extensive history of dating other men. He came out at an early age to his parents who were very accepting and supportive of his gayness. This acceptance served Michael well in that he was proud of being gay, especially at an earlier time when the population was discriminated against. His self-esteem did not suffer from being gay nor did he internalize any homophobia regarding his sexual orientation identity.

When Michael first met Lawrence, he was clearly the more confident of the two. Lawrence had only recently come out and his family was mixed on the issue. In turn, Lawrence tried to limit who he shared his orientation with and stayed away from what he referred to as the "gay scene."

While attending a straight friend's wedding, Lawrence met Michael and was taken by him instantly. The couple soon began a relationship, but quickly ran into trouble. Michael expected that Lawrence would let him take him under his wing and help him to be a proud gay man. However, his unconscious conflict would not allow him to see Michael's unyielding loyalty to his family. Lawrence had different expectations. He hoped that Michael would allow him to move slowly and to hide as much of his gayness as possible from outside. He, however, did not fully acknowledge Michael's need to be true to himself no matter the personal or professional costs.

The couple reported for treatment when they had a huge fight when Lawrence decided to go to a company Christmas party without Michael. He expected Michael to understand his ambivalence about exposing too much of himself as gay, but Michael didn't.

Lesbian Couple

Nicki and Susan have been dating for several months but have yet to live together. Nicki sought therapy for the couple because she wanted to move in together, marry, and to someday have children. Susan came out recently to her family who did not take it well. She feared that she would totally lose them the closer she got to Nicki.

Although she was trying to negotiate a compromise with her family, Nicki was outraged and pressuring Susan to stand up to her parents. But Susan finally had enough and was about to leave Nicki when Nicki suggested trying therapy. It turned out that Susan was happy to have come out when she did, and was proud to be gay, but she was trying to keep her family as well. She expected Nicki to understand her dilemma even though it was clear from the beginning Nicki was more radical about gay advocacy than she was.

Nicki expected Susan to be all in with the gay lifestyle even though she knew from the beginning of their relationship that Susan was too close to her family for this to happen. Nevertheless, Nicki's philosophy was that sometimes gay people had to sacrifice their families to be true to themselves.

More and more couples across the globe are marrying outside of their heritage and when they need treatment, they justifiably expect therapists to be empathic to their plights and to consider their societal, cultural, racial, religious, and sexual differences in a knowledgeable and respectful manner. Every modern-day couples therapist must learn to accept these differences to provide effective treatment. Ignoring them will only be alienating and degrading and exacerbate any problematic conflicts the couples may have with expectations.

References

Abdelmoez, J. W. (2018). Muscles, Moustaches, and Machismo: Narratives of masculinity by Egyptian English-language media professionals and media audiences. *A Journal of Identity and Culture, 9–1*, 197–225.

Allen, T., & Helm, K. (2013). Threats to intimacy for African American couples. In K. Helm & J. Carlson (Eds.), *Love, intimacy, and the African American Couple* (pp. 85–116). Routledge.

Aman, J., Abbas, J., Nurunnabi, & Bano, S. (2019). The relationship of religiosity and marital satisfaction: The role of religious commitment and practices on marital satisfaction among Pakistani respondents. *Behavioral Sciences, 9*, 1–13, doi: 10.3390/bs90300

Anderson, L., & Scherer, Z. (2020, December). U.S. marriages and divorces declined in last 10. years. United States Census Bureau, 2020. Retrieved from www.census.gov/library/stor ies/2020/12/united-states-marriage-and-divorce-rates-declined-last-10-years.html

Atwood, J.D. (2012). Couples and money: The last taboo. *The American Journal of Family Therapy, 40*, 1–19. doi:10.1080/01926187.2011.600674

Baroso, A. (2021). For American couples, gender gaps in sharing household responsibilities persist amid pandemic. Pew Research Center. Retrieved from www.bing.com/search?q= Barroso%2C+A.+(2021

Bar-Tur, I., Ifrah, K., Moore, D., Kamin, S. T., & Lang, F. R. (2018). How do emotional closeness from parents relate to Israeli and German students' life satisfaction Journal of Family Issues, *39*, 3096–3123. https://doi.org/10.1177/0192513X18770213

Bellah, R. (1973). *Emile Durkheim on morality and society*. University of Chicago Press.

Betchen, S. (2018, May). 8 worst reasons people marry: The failure to consider the future of your relationship. www.psychologytoday.com/us/node/1114765/preview

Betts, J. (2022). Egyptian family life today. Retrieved from https://family.lovetoknow.com/ cultural-heritage-symbols/Egyptian-family-life-today

Bhruga, D., & De Silva, P. (2000). Couple therapy across cultures. *Sexual and Relationship Therapy, 15*, 183–192. doi: 10.1080/14681990050010763

Bialik, K. (2017). Key facts about race and marriage, 50 years after Loving v. Virginia. Retrieved from www.pewresearch.org/fact-tank/2017/06/12key-facts-about-race-and-marriage-50-years-after-loving-v-virginia/

Bolotnyy, V. & Emanuel, N. (2022). How unpredictable schedules widen the gender gap. Harvard Business Review. Retrieved from https://hbr.org/2022/07/how-unpredictable-shcedules-widen-the-gender-gap

Borras-Guevara, M.L., & Batres, C., & Perrett, D. I. (2019). Fear of violence among Columbian women is associated with reduced preferences for high-BMI men. *Human Nature, 30*, 341–369. https://doi.org/10/1007/s1210-019-09350-8

Brodie, C. (2019). We need to discuss hyper-masculinity in Israeli culture. 5. Retrieved from https://newvoices.org/2019/09/10/we-need-to-discuss-hyper-masculinity-in-the-Israeli-culture/

Bruk, D. (2019). New study reveals how men and women perceive housework differently. BestLife. Retrieved from www.google.com/search?q=Bruk%2C+D.+(2019)+New+study+ reveals+how+men+and+women+perceive+housework+differently.+BestLife.

Bryant, J. (2022). Women continue to outnumber men in college completion. Best Colleges. Retrieved from www.bestcolleges.com/news/analysis/2021/11/19/women-complete-coll ege-more-than-men/

Camarota, S.A., & Zeigler, K. (2022). Foreign-born population study hits record 46.6 million in January 2022. Center for Immigration Studies. Retrieved from https://cis.org/Camarota/ ForeignBorn-Population-Hits-Record-466-Million-January-2022

Chadda, R. K., & Deb, K. S. (2013). Indian family systems, collectivistic society and psychotherapy. *Indian Journal of Psychiatry, 55*, S299–309. doi: 10.4103/0019-5545.105555. PMID: 23858272; PMCID: PMC3705700.

Chao, R. K. (1994). Beyond parental control and authoritarian parenting style: Understanding Chinese parenting through the cultural notion of training. *Child Development, 65,* 1111–1119.

Cohen-Almagor, R., & Maroshek-Klarman, U. (2022). Gender discrimination in Israel. In A. Tye, J. Carby-Hall, & Z. Góral (Eds.), *Anti-discrimination and employment law: International legal perspectives* (pp. 1–25). Routledge.

Connolly, C. (2012). *Lesbian couples and marriage counseling.* American Counseling Association.

David, P., & Stafford, L. (2015). A relational approach to religion and spirituality in marriage: The role of couple's religious communication in marital satisfaction. *Journal of Family Issues, 36,* 232–249. Htps://doi.org/10.1177/0192513X13485922

Dee, J. (2015). Why Christians is it important for Christians to marry Christians? Uncovering Intimacy. Retrieved from www.uncoveringintimacy.com/why-it-is-improtant-for-christians-to-marry-christians/

Durkheim, E. (1973). Origin of the idea of the totemic principle or mana. In R. Bellah (Ed.), *On morality and society* (pp. 167–186). University of Chicago Press.

Dworkin, s., & Pope, M. (2012). (Eds.). *Casebook for counseling for lesbian, gay, bisexual, and transgendered persons and their families.* American Counseling Association.

European Business Review (2022). Find Columbia wife – Why men want to marry them & how much it will cost. Retrieved from www.europeanbusinessreview.com/find-columibian-wife-why-men-want-to-marry-them-and-how-much-it-costs/

Evans, J., Sahgal, N., Salazar, A. M., Starr, K. J., & Corichi, M. (2022). How Indians view gender roles in families and society. Pew Research Center. Retrieved from www.pewresearch.org/religion/2022/03/02/gender-roles-in-the-family/

Evason, N. (2019). Greek Culture. Cultural Atlas. Retrieved from https://culturalatlas.sbs.com.au.greek.au/greek-culture/greek-culture-family

Expatgroup.co. (2021). Marrying a Columbian: 4 customs to be aware of. Retrieved from https://expatgroup.co/english/expats-in-colombia/marrying-a-colombia-4-customs-to-be-aware-of/

Falconier, M., Randall, A. K., & Bodenmann, G. (2016*). Couples coping with stress: A cross-cultural perspective.* Routledge.

Falicov, C. J. (2014). *Latino families in therapy* (2nd ed.). Guilford.

Fei-Yin Ng, F., & Wei, J. (2020). Delving into the minds of Chinese parents: What beliefs motivate their learning-related practices? *Child Development Perspectives,14,* 61–67 https://doi.org/10.1111/cdep.12358

Ford, A. (2017). Millennial women are conflicted about being breadwinners. Retrieved from Rfinery29: www,refinery29.com/en-us/2017/04/miout-earning-boyfriends-a...

Frost, P., & Meyer, l. (2010). Internalized homophobia and relationship quality among lesbians, gay men, and bisexuals. *Journal of Counseling Psychology, 56,* 97–109. doi:10.1037/a00112844

Fry, R. (2022). Young women are out-earning young men in several U.S. cities. Pew Research Center. Retrieved from www.bing.com/search?q=Fry%2C+R.+%282022%29.

Garbinsky, E., Gladstone, J., Nikolova, H., Olson, J. (2020). Love, lies, and money: Financial infidelity in romantic relationships. *Journal of Consumer Research, 47,* 1–24. https://doi.org/10.1093/jcr/ucz052

Geiger, A. W., & Parker, K. (2018). For women's history month, a look at gender gains-and gaps-in the U.S. Retrieved from Pew Research Center website: www.pewresearch.org/fact-tank/2018/03/15/for-womens-hisotry-month-a-look-

Gonzalez, J. (2020). 10 joys and challenges of having a Columbian partner. Learn More Than Spanish. Retrieved from https://learnmorethanspanish.com/blog/10-joys-and-challenges-of-having-a-columbian-partner/

Hall, E. T. (1990a). *The hidden dimension*. Anchor Books.

Hall, E. T. (1990b). *The silent language*. Anchor Books.

Helm, K., & Carlson, J. (2013). (Eds.). *Love, intimacy, and the African American couple*. Routledge.

Howard, K. (2016). Gay men's relationships: 10 ways they differ from straight relationships. Retrieved from www.huffpost-com/entry/gay-mens-relationships-ten-ways-they-dif fer-from...

Huffpost (2014). Survey reveals which European country cheats most. Retrieved from www. huffpost.com/entry/infidelity-europe_n_4892732

Jewish News of Northern California. (1997). American women who marry Israeli men face a culture clash. Retrieved from https://weekly.com/1997/08/15/american-women-who-marry-israeli-men-face-a-culture-clash/

Jewish Women's Archive (2010). Is intermarriage more likely to end in divorce? Retrieved from https://wa.org/blog/is-intermarriage-more-likely-to-end-in-divorce

Jordan, J., & Carlson, J. (2013). *Creating connection: A relational-cultural approach with couple*s. Routledge.

Karis, T., & Killian, K. (2009). *Intercultural couples: Exploring diversity in intimate relationships*. Routledge.

Kelly, S. (2017). (Ed.), *Diversity in couple and family therapy: Ethnicities, sexualities, and socioeconomics*. Praeger.

Kreuz, R., & Roberts, R. (2017). *Getting through: The pleasures and perils of cross-cultural communication*. MIT Press.

Lee, C. (2015). How to critically use globally discerned case studies in local contexts. In R. Moodley, M. Lengyell, R. Wu, & U. Gielen (Eds.), *International counseling: Case studies handbook* (pp. 3–11). Alexandria, VA: American Counseling Association.

Lee, C., & Park, D. (2013). A conceptual framework for counseling across cultures. In C. Lee and D, Park (Eds.). *Multicultural issues in counseling: new approaches to diversity* (4th ed., pp. 3–12). American Counseling Association.

Lee, E., & Bhuyan, R. (2013). Negotiating within whiteness in cross-cultural clinical encounter. *Social Service Review, 87*, 98–103. doi; 10.1084669919

Lee, E., & Horvath, A. O. (2013). Early cultural dialogues in cross-cultural clin-ical practice. *Smith College Studies in Social Work, 83*, 185–212. doi: 10.1080/ 00377317.2013.8026.39

Lee, E., & Horvath, A.O. (2014). How a therapist responds to cultural versus noncultural dialogues in cross-cultural clinical practice. *Journal of Social Work Practice, 28*, 193–217. doi: 10/1080/026/50533.2013.821104

Liu, L., & Wang, M. (2015). Parenting stress and children's parenting behavior in China: The mediating role of parental psychological aggression. *Journal of Family Psychology, 29*, 20–28. doi.10.1037/fam0000047

Llerena-Quinn, R., & Bacigalupe, G. (2009). Constructions of difference among Latino/ Latina immigrant and non-Hispanic white couples. In T. Karis, and K. Killian (Eds.), *Intercultural couples: Exploring diversity in intimate relationships* (pp. 167–187). Routledge.

MacIver, R. M., & Page, C. H. (1949). *Society: An introductory analysis*. Rinehart.

Madrigal, C. (2013). Columbians in the United States: A study of their well-being. *Advances in Social Work, 14*, 26–48.

Malinowski, B. (2013). *A scientific theory of culture and other essays*. Read Books, Ltd.

Marciano, R. (2019). Childless in a child-centered society. Retrieved from www.jpost.com/ Magazine/Childless-in-a-child-centered-society-582726

Marsella, A. J. & Yamada, A. M. (2010). Culture and psychopathology: Foundations, Issues, Directions. *Journal of Pacific Rim Psychology, 4*, 103–115.

Okasha, T., Elkholy, H., & El-Ghamry, R. (2012). Overview of the family structure in Egypt and its relation to psychiatry. *International Review of Psychiatry, 24*, 162–165. doi: 10.3109/09540261.2012.658030. PMID: 22515467.

Parker, K. (2021). What's behind the growing gap between men and women in college completion? Pew Research Center. Retrieved from www.pewresearch.org/fact-tank/2021/11/08/whats-behind-the-growing-gap-between-men-and-women-in-college-com pletion/

Parsons, T. (1937/1968). *The structure of social action*. (Vol I. 2nd ed.). Free Press.

Pew Research Center (2021). Retrieved from Jewish Americans in 2020: Marriage, families and children. www.pewresearch.org/religion/2012/05/11/marriage-families-and-children/

Rastogi, M. & Thomas, V. (Eds.). (2009). *Multicultural couple therapy*. Sage.

Sahgal, N., & Cooperman, A. (2016). Pew Research Center. Israel's religiously divided society. Retrieved from www.pewresearch.org/religion/2016/03/intergroup-marriage-and-friendship/

Sauerheber, J. D., Hughley, A. W., Wolf, C. P., & Ginn, B. (2020). The relationship among and between marital satisfaction, religious faith, and political orientation. *The Family Journal, 29*, 41–49. https://doi.org/10.1177/1066480720939023

Schaeffer, K. (2019). Among U.S. couples, women do more cooking and grocery shopping than men. Pew Research Center. Retrieved from https://policycommons.net/artifacts/616 594/among-us/1597277/

Semaan, J. (2016). The struggle of the Lebanese man. Human Development Project. Retrieved from https://medium.com/human-development-project/the-struggle-of-the-lebanese-man-4e944e2ee4e6

Shapiro, M. (2007). Money: A therapeutic tool for couples therapy. *Family Process, 46*, 279–291. doi: 10.1111/j.1545-5300.2007.00211.x

Singer, J. (2018). We need to talk about how Israeli men treat American women. Haaretz. Retrieved from www.haaretz.com/us-news/2018-06-18/ty.

Singh, S., & Durso, L. E. (2017). Widespread discrimination continues to shape LGBT people's lives in both subtle and significant ways. Retrieved from www.americanprogress.org/article/widespread-discrimination

Syrda, J. (2019). Spousal relative income and male psychological distress. *Personality and Social Psychology Bulletin*. doi: 10.1177/0146167219883611

Tanap, R. (2019). Why Asian-Americans and Pacific Islanders don't go to therapy. National Association on Mental Illness (NAMI). Retrieved from www.nami.org/Blogs/NAMI-Blog/July-2019/Why-Asian-Americans-and-Pacific-Islanders-Don-t-go-to-Therapy

Tylor, E. B. (1873/2016). *Primitive culture* (Vol. 1). Dover Publications.

United Nations (2022). The fight for gender equality in Lebanon. Human Rights Office of the Commission. Retrieved from www.ohchr.org/enT/2022/05/fight-gender-equality-lebanon

Weber-Gilmore, G., Rose, S., & Rubenstein, R. (2014). The impact of internalized homophobia on outness for lesbian, gay, and bisexual individuals. *The Professional Counselor, 1*, 163–175. doi:10.152/gwv.1.3.163

Wike, R. (2014). French more accepting of infidelity than people in other countries. Pew Research Center. Retrieved from www.pewresearch.org/fact-tank/2014-more-accepting-of-infidelity-tha-peopel-in-other-conutries/

Winkler, I., & Doherty, W. J. (1983). Communication styles and marital satisfaction in Israeli and Arab couples. *Family Process*, *22*, 221–228. doi.1111/j.1545-5300.1983.00221.x

Zaker, B.S., & Boostanipoor, A. (2016). Multiculturalism in counseling and therapy: Marriage and family issues. *International Journal of Psychology and Counseling*, *8*, 53–57. doi: 10.5897/UPC20160388

Section II

Clinical Assessment of Expectations

5 Assessing Couples with Unmet Expectations

The Initial Contact

Assessing unbalanced or unrealistic expectations in couples begins with the initial contact – usually either by telephone or email. I recommend that this be done by telephone because there is a lot you can decipher through live contact that you may not otherwise. For example, a woman called on behalf of her and her husband and, as is my custom, I asked her to briefly describe the chief complaint or presenting problems. A less formal way of asking this is: "What brings you to seek couples therapy?" However, in this case the woman kept talking and refused to let me off the telephone. She insisted on telling me her life story and demanded some immediate advice. When I politely told her that I had prior commitments to honor she became irate and said that I was only interested in getting my fee. She added that if I cared about her, I would allow her to continue speaking. I again explained that I had listened to her quite intently and that I was interested in her story but at that moment I could not accommodate her. I also mentioned that I did not think it was appropriate, or beneficial to her, that I offer any premature interventions before I better understood her case. It was likely that this woman was going to expect an inappropriate amount of energy from me once in treatment and that this might be a replication of the issues in her marriage.

Sometimes a client may call, offer only the symptom, and then immediately ask for advice, as if they expect the therapist to be a self-help columnist. I have experienced this especially when sexual problems are involved because the public tends to view these – with the help of the internet – as behavioral or medical problems with potential quick fixes (see Chapter 6, Treating Couples with Unmet Expectations). These prospective clients often get annoyed if their requests are not honored. In all fairness, some people do not know how therapy works, or if it is distinguishable from "advice," but others do and have their own agenda (e.g., to see if the therapist will treat them as special). Ironically, the therapist who falls for this might find out that the client may not even make an appointment. This often leaves the therapist feeling angry and taken advantage of.

Sometimes a client will make initial contact but end up playing telephone tag with the therapist for weeks. While this might be innocent, it could also be a sign

DOI: 10.4324/9781003359470-7

of unrealistic expectations. For example, some clients get upset if the therapist returns a call but fails to vigorously pursue them even though they fail to return the therapist's call. It is as if the client expects the therapist to want them badly enough to make them a priority.

It is quite common for clients to tell you upon initial contact that they expect you to bend the rules for them. For example, you might bill once a month but to expedite reimbursements from their insurance company a couple may try to negotiate with you to get them the receipts after every session. A client requested special treatment and acted as if he deserved it because he agreed to be my client. He implied that I probably needed the business so badly that I would do anything for him to secure it.

While this is rare compared to the previous examples, some clients expect you to supply them with letters of support before you have even gotten to know them. These letters may be at the behest of their attorneys for a legal issue, or to help them to manipulate certain institutional rules. For example, during our initial telephone conversation a prospective female client told me that she and her new husband were in the process of filing a civil suit against her ex-husband and that they expected a letter of support within four sessions. While this would be annoying to most therapists, at least she did warn rather than surprise me with it after the third or fourth session, which is all too common.

Couples may call to request a letter regarding something that is completely out of my area of expertise. Some have demanded a letter from me addressed to their employer for the purpose of allowing them to bring a pet to work or on an airplane. It never fails that every time I refuse these requests the couple gets mad. They do so even if it might put my license in jeopardy.

Therapists of all levels of training and experience ask me if they should continue to call a client who has disappeared or "ghosted" them. Some want to write the client a letter or send an email to find out what happened. In my experience, most of the time this is about the therapist's anxiety. They may worry that they have hurt the client's feelings, made a mistake in treatment, not worked as hard as they should have, or that the client does not like them. These therapists expect too much from themselves.

Too many therapists overlook the dynamics of the initial contact either because their first concern is getting the couple in for treatment or because they want the case badly enough to ignore any signs that the treatment process will be rough. I always tell my students and supervisees that nothing is free and if it looks too good to be true, it is. I stress never to be desperate. I let them know that the initial contact is a snapshot of how the treatment process will go. Therefore, if the couple expect a lot before actual treatment begins, they will expect more during it.

Although this should be reiterated in the first session, the initial contact is a good time for the therapist to set boundaries and limits with the couple (Doherty, 2002; Weeks & Fife, 2014). The couples therapist should be gentle but firm and make clear what the terms of the treatment are and stick to them. Not all couples are the same: some are very flexible and easy to please; others are impossible to please. In dealing with couples with conflicts around expectations, it is especially important to maintain boundaries because they are more prone to testing them. Fees should be set and consistent, including how the therapist deals with missed sessions and receipts offered.

There are couples who – because of their unbalanced conflicts with expectations – expect too little, but they rarely pose a problem for the couples therapist if the therapist keeps their best interests at heart. However, in these cases sometimes the therapist must protect them from themselves. For example, one couple was referred to me by their attorney even though it was clear they could not afford treatment with me. With their permission, I called the lawyer and explained to him that I feared the couple would get into financial trouble if they saw me. Both he and the couple expected me to take the case but I thought it would do more harm than good and so I referred them to a clinic that charged on a sliding scale. The couple seemed nice but had some trouble standing up to their lawyer and protecting themselves. They expected him to make the right decisions for them and in this case, his preference was not in their best interests.

Another couple called from New York City in need of couples therapy. This was pre-pandemic, and online treatment was not yet available. I refused the couple for several reasons that would protect all of us. I was sure that it would exhaust the couple to drive over two hours a week to get to my office and that this would interfere in therapeutic continuity. And I knew several competent couples therapists in New York City that they would have been happy with. I was also not sure that I could see them legally given I did not hold a license to practice in New York at the time.

Although the couple protested and told me that they were happily willing to make the drive, I decided instead to give them a few referrals in the city. Most couples like these are setting themselves up to fail or to not get their needs met. I did not want to feed into their unbalanced conflict with expectations.

Now that most therapists are treating couples online, barring licensing issues we can see couples from other states. I have received initial contacts from couples in Oklahoma, Texas, Kansas, New Orleans, Florida, California, and from some foreign countries like Africa, England, India, and Pakistan, to name a few. But licensing and liability issues aside, I keep in mind whether a couple's expectations are realistic or potentially sabotaging before agreeing to treat them.

The First Session

It is vital for the couples therapist to *join* with the couple to establish a working relationship. Aponte (2017) wrote: "The first task of couple therapy is to gain trust and partnership of the clients, the foundation of the therapeutic relationship" (p. 11). It is best if some pleasantries are initially exchanged; however, Aponte claims the couples therapist would be best to find "…something in themselves that they can identify personally with the client to the point of empathy, even as they remain well-grounded in the differentiated self" (p. 12). Especially since the therapist has already spoken to one partner, it is important to relate, as soon as possible, to the non-initialing partner for the sake of balance.

The formal assessment process usually takes one to two sessions, preferably with both partners present, although the couples therapist should remain open to receiving additional information throughout the treatment process. Some couples therapists prefer to send a couple a pre-treatment assessment evaluation such as the Enhanced Gottman Assessment Test (Gottman & Gottman, 2022). These instruments can be helpful especially if they help to assess the expectations of each partner. Questions might include those assessing aspirations both personal and professional, values, life goals, and how much support they expect from a partner.

Because the MCT model is an integrative approach which combines psycho-analytic and systemic concepts with the basic principles of sex therapy, I use the genogram as the assessment tool of choice. The genogram allows the couples therapist to easily record each partner's history and specific familial influences, sexual data, and relational dynamics – especially conflicts with expectations (Bowen, 1978; DeMaria et al., 2017; Gambescia et al., 2021; Hof & Berman, 1986).

By drawing two genograms, the couples therapist can then proceed to ask each partner questions which are relevant to the couple's case, and to record the respective information on each genogram. Unfortunately, couples are notorious for avoiding this process by fighting or by obsessing about their symptoms.

When a couple constantly is on transmit and prevents the clinician from speaking or offering any constructive interventions, this can be interpreted as: 1) a glimpse of their day-to-day dynamic; and 2) as a defense to protect their shared conflict against an assault by the therapist. The couples therapist must be assertive and stop the bickering long enough to get the information needed to help the couple. It is valuable to see a client's real-life dynamic in the treatment room. But if it lingers and blocks the therapist from obtaining significant information, the therapist should let the partners know that they cannot be helped by blocking clinical inquiries.

In the MCT model, the therapist is always looking for signs that an unbalanced conflict with expectations is predominant in the couple's dynamics and in turn their symptoms. Some signs are blatant, but others are quite subtle. Regardless, the therapist must be sure to give proper credence to these hints because they offer valuable information that the clinician can use whenever the time is right to confront the client about their conflict with expectations.

The first example that comes to mind is when a couple shows up late to the first session and expects the therapist to allow them full-session time, or to pay a partial fee even though they have used the clinician's entire hour. One way to lessen the chance of this happening is to immediately set the structure of the treatment (Weeks & Fife, 2014).

Doherty (2002) claimed that beginning couples therapists have trouble providing couples with appropriate structure. But even so, couples with expectation issues will often breach rules and insist that the therapists do the same. It is too early for the therapist to contribute a breach of this kind to a conflict with unmet expectations, but this information should be registered by the therapist for later use after more data is gathered. It will then be easier and more effective for the therapist to make his/her case to the couple.

Another common example is when a couple expects the therapist to do the work for them. Sometimes this may manifest in pressuring the therapist to do all the talking. For example, a female client let me know that because she and her husband were paying me, she expected me to start the sessions and to maintain the verbal flow. While I do think the couples therapist does need a game plan, he/she should not be more motivated to help the couple change than they are. This will only lead to a poor prognosis.

There are also couples that expect a solution to their problems immediately after the initial session. This is also a defense against real change. Couples are anxious to get rid of their pain. But most couples have been living with pain for some time and to expect a quick fix is unrealistic. While this may be a sign of entitlement, it could also serve as a defense to be dissatisfied with the therapist and to prematurely terminate treatment.

The couples therapist cannot prevent termination if the couple insists on ending treatment. But I usually let the couple know that there will be no gain without pain, and that pressuring me to cure them might not be in their best interests. I may also tell a couple that although we have the same goals for treatment in mind, we might not have the same way of reaching them. Often this calms them, especially if they have no premeditated intention of dropping out.

Treadway (2020) wrote: "Couples often come into therapy at war with each other and like lawyers or siblings, they usually have prepared briefs to present in front of the judge or the parent" (p. 20). The point, of course, is to get the therapist to choose sides. While a client may try to accomplish this via an email or text prior to the first session, he/she may also attempt it in the beginning of treatment as well.

Because the art of couples therapy lies in the delicate balancing of the couple, the therapist must avoid siding with one partner over the other at all costs (Wachtel, 2017). While this is usually difficult, if a parent has enabled a partner, he/she might have an expectation that they will be favored in the treatment process. This could be loosely referred to as a transference, a concept that will be dealt with in Chapter 7, The Therapist's Unmet Expectations. If such a situation gets too out of control, the therapist can explain to the demanding partner that alienating the other will only lead to a poor therapeutic prognosis.

If, after the first meeting, the therapist is bombarded by lengthy emails or texts about the session, it is a sign that the partner sending these is trying to control the treatment or to sway the therapist's loyalty (Betchen, 2022). Some clients expect the therapist to respond to these messages no matter how often they are told that this can threaten the welfare of the treatment process. In fact, it would not be unusual if a client or couple became enraged with the therapist for setting limits with them. All that the therapist can do in this situation is to set the limits in a professional manner and hope for the best. If the client or couple is too dysfunctional to adhere to the rules of the treatment process, they might not be well enough to take advantage of the treatment process.

There are some couples that seek treatment but insist that the therapist use a model that they have read a book about, seen on the internet, or had a friend recommend. I have had more than one couple come to the first session with a paperback on a particular model and request that I use the approach in the book.

A male client told me that he expected that I read the book and apply the author's methods. He stated that it was part of my job to do so. I gently told him that I was familiar with this model and that my approach incorporated similar aspects, but if he would prefer someone trained specifically in it, I would refer him. Some of these people unconsciously use another therapist's model as a context for their conflict with expectations. If, however, sabotaging behavior and negative transferences are under control, the couples therapist can get around this resistance and smoothly proceed to conduct an assessment using the genogram.

Although rare, a couple will present that are incompatible with MCT and be better off seeking a behavioral treatment approach. Rather than try and convince them that your model is best, it is important for the therapist to accept that therapy is not a "one size fits all" process, and a couple may in fact be better suited for a different treatment method. In this case an appropriate referral is merited.

As mentioned in previous work (Berman, 1982; Betchen, 2022; Betchen & Davidson, 2018), some questions are better asked in an individual format. For example, if the couples therapist suspects an ongoing affair or prior abuse. I recommend that after the first session or two, the therapist sees each partner alone at least once to obtain the more delicate information. While this may put the therapist in the awkward position of having to hold a secret, at least the therapist will be fully aware of what is needed to better treat the couple. The therapist should be aware, however, that some partners are intimidated by this gesture – usually those who fear the loss of the relationship most. These individuals may be too anxious to be split up out of concern that something may come out that is irreparable. The therapist should calm the anxious partner but make no promises that all will end well. Sometimes, for example, a partner will tell the therapist that he no longer loves his wife, and he has wanted to leave for years. The therapist must hold this information in confidence but can convince the partner to expose it for the ultimate good of the couple. If the client refuses, a referral for individual treatment should be made. Rather than breach confidence, the therapist can then make the general statement that: "couples therapy is not recommended at this time."

Some couples feel that an assessment of the family of origin is simply a way to blame their parents for their issues. The therapist can assure them, however, that the purpose is not to denigrate parents, but to examine any influences that might have led to the couple's symptoms. The therapist can reiterate that each partner will be held accountable for their respective contributions to their relationship problems.

Questions for the Genogram

To conduct an accurate and extensive assessment, the therapist needs to gather sufficient background on the couple. Rather than burden the reader here, I will only offer a general list of questions that were compiled from two previous sources (Betchen, 2022, pp. 57–73; Betchen & Davidson, 2018, pp. 62–66), which can be consulted for additional details. All questions are preferably asked of each partner when they are both present, although, as mentioned, it may be appropriate to ask some of the more sensitive questions – denoted by asterisks – in individual sessions (Berman, 1982).

What do you see as the major reason for contacting me?
When did you first start having this problem?
Have you ever sought treatment for this problem before?
Have you ever experienced this problem in a previous relationship?
Do you have siblings?
Are you in contact with your siblings?
What is the relationship status of your siblings?
Do any of your siblings have the same problem you do?
How would you describe each of your parent's personalities when growing up?
What did each of your parents do for a living?
How would you describe your parents' relationship?
Did your parents ever separate or divorce?
Did one of your parents always seem to be upset with the other?
Did you and your parents share the same or similar interests, political and
*   religious values, or cultural backgrounds?*
Did your parents approve of your relationship?
Did you favor a parent or did one favor you?
Did your parents talk about sex when you were a child?
What role did you play growing up in your family?
Do you have any medical conditions?
Do you take any medications?
At what age did you lose your virginity?
Have you ever experienced abuse of any kind?*
Were you ever exposed to anything sexually provocative?*
Do you masturbate?*
Do you fantasize?*
Do you watch pornography and if so, how often and what kind?*
Do you have any paraphilias or fetishes?*
What type or form of sexual activity excites you the most?
Can you achieve orgasm?
Are you physically attracted to your partner?*
Are you sexually satisfied with your partner?
Did you ever consider having sex with someone of the same sexual orientation?*

How often would you like to have sex?
Can you give me a detailed picture of your last sexual experience?
Do you have a sexually exclusive relationship? *
How long did you and your partner date before you formed an exclusive relationship?
If you had a honeymoon, how would you describe it?
To your knowledge have there ever been any outside relationships or affairs? *
Do you and your partner share the same or similar interests, political and religious values, and cultural backgrounds?
Do you have any children? If so, what are their ages and gender identity and orientation?
If you have children, what roles do they play in your family?

The next set of questions were designed to assess a couple's conflict with expectations and can be added to the general list above as the therapist sees fit. In my clinical experience, it saves time and speeds up the assessment process if the couples therapist learns to ask questions that are specifically aimed at assessing a couple's expectations. The therapist will naturally alter these questions depending on the context of the couple's chief complaint. Last, because this is an integrative model, note that questions regarding the couple's sexual life arc also included to better assess unmet sexual expectations.

What did you expect from your partner once you became seriously involved or married?
This question is asked of both partners, and it would be good to ask it right after the couple announces the presenting symptom. From this answer the therapist can ascertain what was expected, at least on a conscious level, and to assess whether it was within reasonable expectations. If not realistic, a conflict was probably the motivating factor for this choice of partner at the onset. For example, a young woman told me that she expected that the man she married would be able to financially support her if she stopped working and decided to have children. While this in of itself is not an unrealistic expectation, the man she was planning to marry was from a family of modest means, he had dropped out of college, and was currently unemployed. His prospects were limited. If the woman had said that feeling loved was of far greater importance to her than money, this would have been more congruent with her boyfriend's potential, and she would therefore have a greater chance of fulfilling her expectations.

Could you see any problems that might have prevented you from getting what you want in the relationship?
This is an all-important question because the answer may disclose if either partner was conscious of the fact that their expectations would never be fulfilled. The more obvious the blockage, the greater the odds that a conflict is a

factor. Some people have told me that although they recognized the struggle ahead, they relished a challenge. But most do not seem to grasp the size of the challenge until they are already engaged with it. For example, a young woman insisted on marrying a young man with a potentially fatal autoimmune disorder despite her parents' warnings. Because the disease could be slow moving, however, the young woman felt that she had made the right decision. But as time went on the woman's husband became sicker and less mobile causing her to feel trapped. She said she never expected that he would become so incapacitated.

If you answered "yes" to the preceding question, then why did you choose to stay in the relationship?
Clients do not know the answer to this question because the truth is hidden by the unconscious to protect their conflict with expectations. Nonetheless, the question is a valuable one, in part because it encourages couples to think conflict. Most often, partners will tell me they stay because they are still in love, or because of the children, or because of finances, or out of guilt. Some adamantly take the stand that they will not make a move, and yet challenge the therapist to help them feel content in their dilemma – which is extremely difficult to accomplish.

Could you identify any limitations in your partner that might make it difficult to get what you want in the relationship?
This question is like the preceding questions but more specific. The answer will help the therapist to see if the client has any insight into the limitations of the partner they have chosen. To highlight a conflict, it sometimes can help the therapist to reframe a question previously asked.

Were you abused or neglected in your family of origin?
Being mistreated can lead to expecting too much of others. It is as if an entitlement is created that can lead to a lifetime of feeling owed. Others, however, may react differently to the same experience. These people may feel that they are not deserving and in turn develop exceptionally low expectations.

Was one or more siblings favored over you by either parent?
When siblings are favored, the less favored one may internalize the belief that they do not deserve better. If the people who are supposed to love you unconditionally (e.g., parents) fail to do so, it is hard to see yourself as worthy of such love from anybody. These individuals may question whether they are loveable at all. For example, a man was recruited by a brokerage firm specifically because he possessed a certain talent. And while he was flattered and felt important, he quickly sabotaged his career and was fired because of some blatantly risky business decisions he made. The man revealed that he could never please his hypercritical parents who always favored his older brother and sister. He thought that as the youngest sibling, he was a mistake and perceived as a burden by his parents.

When it came to your needs, did you receive mixed messages from one or both parents?

Ambivalence can lead to conflict. For example, some children are labeled "mistakes" in their families of origin. This is usually the oldest or first child or the youngest or last child. Often parents do not realize that they transmit conflicting messages about having these children because they may have not been planned for. The difference between this question and the preceding one, however, is that in the example above, the man's parents were not ambivalent. They made it clear to their son that he was unwanted.

Were you used to getting your needs met in your past intimate relationships?

This can tell the therapist if there is a pattern in intimate relationships of not having one's expectations met. Many people react negatively when asked about their dating history. They think it is irrelevant to their current issues. However, people tend to replicate relationship difficulties and choose the same type of person repeatedly. In this case it would be partners who cannot or will not meet their needs.

While defenses like denial can keep a conflict in place and foster replication, it may sometimes be disguised by context. For example, if a woman grew up in a family with an alcoholic father it would not be a surprising that she chose an alcoholic to marry. However, if she moves on to marry a second time, and is hyperaware of avoiding an alcoholic, she may unconsciously marry a different kind of addict and still not get her marital expectations fulfilled. Once again, she will be second fiddle to whatever addiction her new mate has.

How does your partner react when asked to do something for you?

The answer to this question can tell the therapist how cooperative or resistant partners are and whether there is any interest in meeting relational expectations. Another way of asking this question is whether either partner is investing much of anything to better the relationship. If not, this can certainly be a sign of a conflict. For example, some people refuse to make even the slightest effort to please their respective partner. A man seemed to have the hardest time buying a birthday card for his wife or remembering their anniversary. His wife could not get him to give her even the minimum of compliments. He acted as if the marriage was a depressive container that he simply had to live in, like his family of origin.

If you told your partner what you needed sexually would this be taken seriously?

Same as the preceding question, the answer here tells the therapist if the partner is willing to meet the other's expectations but this time in the context of sexuality. The most common sexual problems presented in treatment is that of low libido. Usually, one partner has no interest in sex and the other does. Low sexual desire or arousal can be caused by many things, but one reason is that one partner is in conflict about their chosen mate. In this way, both partners fail to get their sexual needs met.

Do you think your parents were satisfied with each other?

This tells if the unmet expectations were chronic and yet unattended to in each partner's family of origin. Many people can live with deprivation and replicate it in their present relationships. They are used to not having their expectations met and in many cases are role-modeling their parents' dismal dynamic.

Do you think that your parents tried to please one another?

This is a reframe of the preceding question but more specific. The answer to the question may help to identify any patterns of unmet expectations that each partner may be role modeling in the present. There are some cases in which a child or young adult has witnessed parents who have completely neglected each other, and others where one parent tried hard to please the other but to no avail. Children notice these disparities in the family of origin and may replicate the dynamic in their relationships. Often the parent who tries harder to meet the other's needs is pitied by the child well into adulthood. This may lead to marrying someone who cannot meet a partner's needs but merits pity.

Can you identify something that one parent might have wanted from the other but could not get?

This question concerns a chronic, specific point of contention. It is not unusual, for example, for one parent to complain about the same thing repeatedly, such as a lack of affection. Growing up in this environment, an individual may not be able to avoid unconsciously replicating this dynamic in their adult relationships.

Did you have parents that you could rely on consistently for emotional and financial support?

This gives an indication as to whether a partner's expectations were met unconditionally, albeit appropriately. This background is more likely to promote security than an unruly conflict about expectations.

Did your parents praise you for your accomplishments as a child and young adult?

Appropriate praise is less likely to result in an internal conflict with expectations. While unearned praise may produce spoiled children, appropriate reward for a job well done will not lead to a problematic conflict around expectations. A woman reported to treatment because she felt that her husband did not pay enough attention to her. While this man was indeed a self-contained personality, his wife was extremely cute as a little girl, a beautiful and popular teenager, and a model as an adult. Her parents recognized her attributes and constantly told her how incredible she was: "A perfect gift from God." As a result, when this woman walks into a room, she expects heads to turn; in fact, she would become quite angry and disappointed if this did not happen. Her husband saw her attributes but could not keep up with her needs. Of course, this begs the question: Why would such an introverted, self-contained man marry someone who needs so much attention? The answer lies in a conflict with expectations.

Do you think your parents are proud of the adult you turned into?
This is a similar but more specific question than the preceding one. If parents openly and appropriately praise their child, that child will be less likely to develop a conflict with expectations.

Was there a particular incident involving your parents that disappointed you?
There may have been "one" significant incident that led to a conflict around expectations. For example, a male elementary school student won the school spelling bee. To the young boy it was a huge accomplishment and one that was unexpected given the child was a mediocre student. As the competition increased to the next level, the child's father attended the competition dressed in a t-shirt and pants with paint stains. The child was embarrassed, especially when his teacher made an issue of it. The student expected his father to dress appropriately. When he had his own children, he made sure that he wore a suit and tie to their events. He also expected to be treated equally by others and was quick to anger if he perceived that someone was critical of his social standing.

Did you experience any traumas or shocking incidents in your family of origin or life in general?
As discussed in a previous section, traumatic experiences can lead to internal conflict with expectations in later life. For example, a man's father suffered a fatal heart attack on Christmas morning when his son was a pre-teen. In turn, as an adult the man was in conflict about whether to celebrate Christmas, as well as any other holidays, for years.

Can you identify anything personally or professionally that you have been unable to accomplish or achieve?
The answer to this question allows the therapist to determine whether there is a pattern of unmet expectations that cut across different contexts. It is evidence that a conflict is internalized and pervasive. For example, a young wife with low sexual drive who abstained from having sex with her husband inadvertently informed me that her husband never gets what he wants in life. She specifically mentioned that he can never seem to please his parents and is frequently passed over for promotions at work. She described him as the kind of guy who works hard to get an A but usually misses it by a point or two.

Do you consider yourself assertive when it comes to getting your needs met?
Sometimes you can get what you want if you make your expectations clear. However, some are so confounded by their conflict that they cannot even identify their needs. Others know what they want but are so paralyzed by their conflict that they cannot verbalize their expectations and desires. Nevertheless, both types of people are quite capable of settling for less in their relationships and life in general.

Do you ever feel guilty when you achieve something or when you are complimented?

A conflict can employ guilt to preserve itself. It does so by making one feel terrible when they do get an expectation met. For example, I treated a young man who earned a modest income. But after winning the lottery he expressed guilt and contemplated giving his fortune away to family members and friends. He told me that he was so disturbed that he did not think he could sleep at night knowing that he had so much money and others were starving. This made sense to me because when he would receive an accolade from outsiders as a child, his parents reminded him to stay humble. "Do not get too big for your britches," they would warn.

Interactional Styles

Aside from gathering evidence with the genogram, the couples therapist must keep a sharp eye out for certain interactional styles of communication that may or may not support a conflict with expectations. This is no easy task because partners may express their expectations in a *symmetrical* way or in the same manner and a *complementary* way or in a contrasting manner (Lederer & Jackson, 1968). The following is a list of both symmetrical and complementary styles and the problems they may pose in the treatment process.

Symmetrical Styles

It is hard for the couples therapist to work effectively with two partners in a *symmetrical* relationship. By constantly challenging and fighting with each other they can more easily engage the therapist to feel each other's outrage and to become entangled in their symmetrical struggle. While this is usually unconscious, the couple wish the therapist to feel as they do, and in turn, block the therapist from being able to move the treatment forward. The following three symmetrical styles are addressed: 1) *The confrontational–confrontational couple*; 2) *The elusive–elusive couple*; and 3) *The bickering–bickering couple*.

The Confrontational–Confrontational Couple

Some partners are direct with each other about what they expect from their relationships, though they still might unconsciously sabotage these expectations from being fulfilled. The therapist will not have to work too hard to get a clear picture of the chief complaint. What these individuals claim to be their main concerns is usually an accurate depiction of what is going on. For example, Jane said plainly that she expected more affection from her husband, Bill. Even though she unconsciously sabotaged this expectation from being fulfilled, she was on target about what was lacking in her relationship. That is, Bill was not a very affectionate mate.

A male client, Lance, made it clear throughout treatment that the only problem he had in marriage was that his wife, Ginny, no longer had intercourse with him. And while he stubbornly refused treatment for a chronic case of erectile disorder (ED), he was not wrong that this was the couple's primary symptom, and that Ginny could have refrained from enabling his ED by consistently criticizing his sexual prowess.

The direct couple may seem harsh or too confrontational at times, but they are usually clear about their desired expectations. Sometimes a couple with this interactional style may be taught to address each other in a less offensive manner, but at the very least there will be less confusion about how they feel. This topic is discussed in Chapter 7, Treating Couples with Unmet Expectations.

The Elusive–Elusive Couple

The elusive couple makes it next to impossible for the couples therapist to pin down their expectations. Their unconscious *modus operandi* is to confuse the therapist and themselves so that their conflict remains intact. Towards this end, they may employ several techniques: 1) present a host of symptoms that serve to overwhelm and thus paralyze the therapist; 2) act as if they are not exactly sure why they need treatment; 3) act as if they can never seem to recall what might have triggered an argument; 4) feign confusion about what the therapist is trying to convey; 5) claim they have no idea what their significant other wants; 6) consistently raise the bar so that their needs can never be met; and 7) remain passive in treatment as if they have no control over their relationship process.

It is certainly not unusual for a therapist with this type of couple to conduct treatment for several months and still have no handle on the case. And no wonder... this process is like wrestling with a ghost. Hal and Fern presented for treatment but could not decide on their chief complaint. Both partners attributed their marital woes to a variety of issues and immediately began to shift from symptom to symptom, refusing to spend enough energy on any of them to be helped.

After observing this dynamic for several minutes, and trying to slow the couple down, they responded by telling me that there was so much for me to learn about them and that they needed to get it all out. But much of the information seemed unnecessary and redundant. This would be a hard enough case for an experienced therapist, but it could destroy the confidence level of an inexperienced therapist. One final thought: When Hal and Fern gave me permission to speak with their former therapist, the therapist told me that she did not know what was going on with the couple. She wished me luck.

The Bickering–Bickering Couple

There are some couples who are always on the offensive. They take turns attacking each other and pointing out the ways they did not get what they wanted. It is like a scene from the play by Edward Albee, "Who's Afraid of Virginia

Woolf." Partners take turns jabbing at one another, and sometimes in the most brutal way possible. This may range from name calling to sarcastic snipping at one another. There seems to be no area, no matter how personal, that is exempt from attack. This constant offensive serves to block any productive discussion about expectations and in turn, maintains the couple's conflict.

Rather than focus specifically on what they wanted from each other, a newly married couple, Tom and Lisa, incessantly traded barbs without allowing me to intervene. And if I forced my way into their dynamic, they gave me a second or two and immediately picked up where they left off without acknowledging a word that I said. Tom and Lisa took turns attacking each other's parents, friends, handling of finances, hygiene, and dress. Eventually, the couple began to up the ante by taking turns graphically criticizing each other's body parts and sexual techniques. It was a relentless process.

The bickering vs. bickering couple can be volatile at times and the couples therapist may have trouble breaking up their style long enough for any productive work to occur. The therapist might need to temporarily stop the treatment and warn the couple that they will get nowhere if they continue to fight; that under these conditions they are wasting their time and money. If this intervention fails, however, it might be more appropriate to refer each partner for individual therapy to better prepare them for couples therapy.

Complementary Styles

As mentioned, couples may present for treatment with contrasting or *complementary* styles. And while symmetrical couples are hard enough to work with, a complementary couple adds a different complexity. For example, their communication is often poor because they have diverse ways to express themselves. A complementary couple is more likely to be even more difficult for the couples therapist to treat in part, because one or both partners often compete for the therapist's attention and favor in the treatment. This way, the couple are better able to unbalance the treatment and risk premature termination. But the ultimate objective is to protect the couple's underlying conflict from any clinical challenges that might better treat the couple's troubled conflict. There are three predominant contrasting combinations: 1) *the confrontational–elusive couple*; 2) *the bickering–elusive couple*; and 3) the *bickering–confrontational couple*.

The Confrontational–Elusive Couple

If a confrontational partner and an elusive partner join, at first, they may seem as if they formed the perfect match – each partner complements the other. The confrontive partner may assert him/herself to outsiders for the good of the couple and the elusive partner may avoid an altercation with outsiders that might protect the couple from further turmoil. For example, Jill, the confrontational partner, was not afraid of sending undercooked food back at a restaurant or to confront an aggravating neighbor or family member. In this sense she was not shy about going after what she wanted. Ray, however, the elusive partner, found this level of assertiveness difficult and chose simply to eat the uncooked food or to ignore unruly outsiders. He would sacrifice his expectations and act at times as if he had none.

While the match between Jill and Ray may seem like it was made in heaven, troubles may ensue when each partner plays their respective roles within the relationship. That is, when Jill comes on too strong for Ray, he may run from her or respond in a passive-aggressive manner. It is an interactional style that is reminiscent of the pursuer–distancer dynamic (Betchen, 2005; Fogarty, 1979).

The Bickering–Elusive Couple

The bickering–elusive style is like the confrontational–elusive combination. The difference is that although the bickering partner may be confrontational, he/she relentlessly complains or badgers the elusive partner to get his/her needs met. True to a conflict with expectations, however, this behavior only serves to chase the elusive partner further away. For example, Adele badgered her husband Jesse over every little thing that she wanted him to do for her. Whether it was going grocery shopping or fixing a broken door in the house, it always seemed to Jesse as if Adele had something for him to do and she pestered him until he did it.

Jesse claimed that this would not be so bad if, after he completed a task, he could rest. But he said that Adele always had a new job waiting; and that she would become increasingly angry if he did not complete each task immediately. This was, in fact, a common way for Adele *not* to get her needs met because the more she badgered Jesse, the more he procrastinated.

The Bickering–Confrontational Couple

This combination is potentially explosive because the bickering partner will often badger the confrontive partner. If the confrontational partner holds his/her feelings in for too long a time to spare an argument, there may be an explosion coming that the bickering partner might not have prepared for. While the bickering partner may be confrontational, the reverse is not necessarily true. One can be confrontational when needed but the bickering partner is far more relentless.

Patty badgered her husband Tom even though Tom could be aggressive when he needed to be. And while he gave Patty the benefit of the doubt because he was better able to put things behind him, when Patty would focus on something that bothered her, she could not let it go. She was far more obsessive than Tom and would bring up things that he might have done years ago. When this occurred, Tom would explode and shut Patty down. In truth, Tom would often apologize for any behavior Patty deemed bad or disappointing, but this never met Patty's needs, and she would continue to badger Tom into intermittent explosions which caused him great stress. Tom believed that Patty was solely responsible for his high blood pressure. At one point in the treatment, he claimed that she was unconsciously trying to kill him.

Armed with information gathered by the genogram, and a knowledge of the interactional styles of couples, the couples therapist can proceed to conduct an extensive assessment. The following two cases illustrate the assessment phase.

Assessing Latisha and Lucas (See Figure 5.1)

The Initial Contact

Latisha contacted me via telephone to request treatment for her and her husband of eight years, Lucas. Latisha was a 42-year-old stay-at-home spouse and Lucas was a 66-year-old attorney. A Black couple, this was the second marriage for Lucas and the first for Latisha. Lucas had two teenage children from his first marriage and Latisha had one, a 10-year-old daughter from a long-term relationship.

For the chief complaint, Latisha reported that the couple were fighting frequently over the children. She claimed that her husband was very territorial and separated what was his from other family members. Latisha said this was rude and uncaring and it especially hurt her daughter, who was not used to this behavior. For example, Lucas would buy himself a pizza and become enraged if her daughter took a slice without asking permission from him.

Latisha also complained that Lucas treated money the same way. What was his, was his, and not a family asset. Latisha said Lucas was like this with his first wife and this was the reason for his divorce. She said that his selfish behavior upsets his children as well, but they are used to it and do not take it as rejection. She made it clear that she would not allow Lucas to bully her or her daughter.

Latisha admitted that before she met Lucas, she was a struggling single parent who didn't have any financial help from her estranged ex-boyfriend. When she started dating Lucas, she claimed that he was generous and acted interested in being a father to her daughter. This was what she expected of him. When I asked her what she thinks Lucas expected of her she said that he wanted a pretty woman on his arm, especially given their age discrepancy. She also said that Lucas wants her to resume having sex with him – something she has stopped providing out of annoyance.

When I inquired as to how Lucas felt about therapy, she said they agreed on it and that he was looking forward to registering his complaints about the marriage. I instantly liked Latisha and I got a good feeling about this couple. I believe they had integrity and would abide by the therapeutic structure.

The First Session

Lucas started off the session by agreeing with Latisha's view of the chief complaint. However, in doing so he added that he was especially upset with the lack

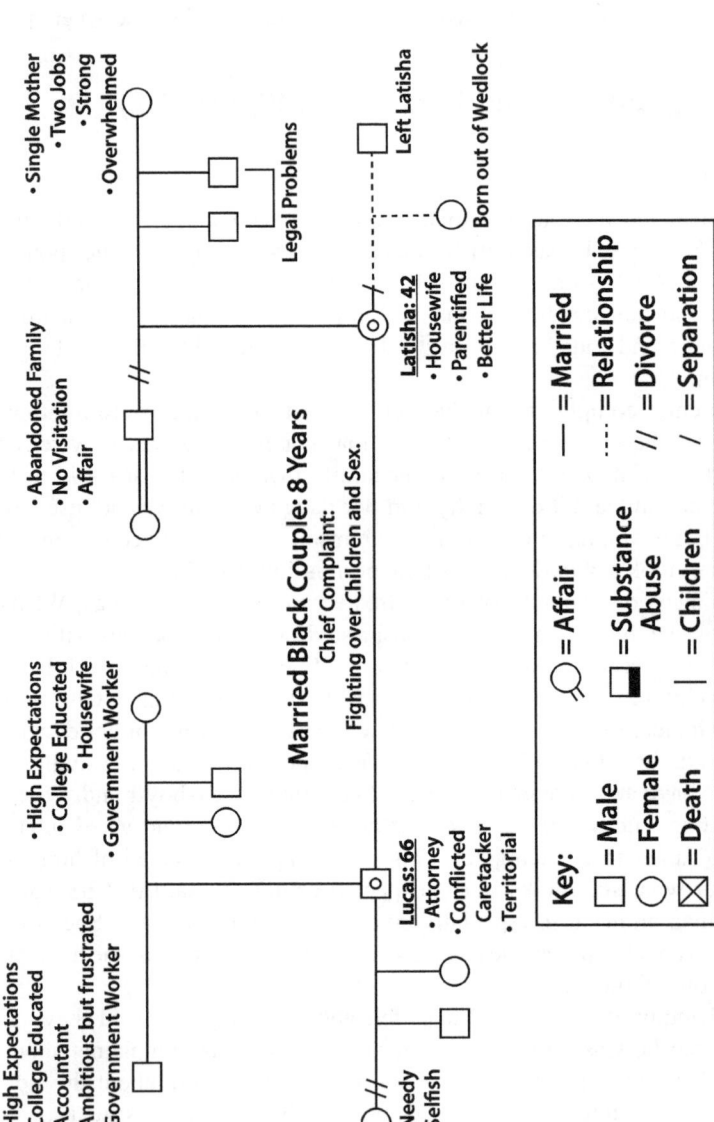

Figure 5.1   Latisha and Lucas.

of affection and her refusal to have sex with him. He said that their pre-marriage sex life was "great" but soon after marriage Latisha began to pull away.

Lucas did admit that he could be territorial with his things but that was in response to Latisha's difficulty setting limits with any of the children. Latisha countered that she always had a strong sex drive, but that Lucas has worn her down with his selfish behavior. She claimed that she still found him attractive, but that she was angry and disappointed. She said that life with him was "conditional." She reiterated that she initially saw Lucas as a loving, giving man but soon he became cheap, selfish, and vindictive. It was apparent that this couple was caught in a vicious cycle: The more selfish Latisha perceived Lucas the more she distanced from him sexually and otherwise. This in turn would cause Lucas to become even more irate and nagging.

Given this was a very bright and articulate couple, it was easy to see that both had expectations that were not being fulfilled. What they initially expected was not what they were currently getting. Latisha expected Lucas to be unconditionally giving. She especially thought this way because he took on a poor single parent at his late age. Latisha said that Lucas did not need to do this and that only a good-hearted person would consider it.

Lucas did not mind taking care of Latisha's daughter, but he expected more of her than he did his children. Lucas claimed that what really attracted him to Latisha was youth, beauty, and her high sex drive. He said that he was tired of dating women his age because he did not find them as attractive or exciting.

The Genogram

An extensive sexual history revealed nothing remarkable. Both partners functioned well sexually in past relationships and did so in their relationship until each began to feel betrayed by the other. There was no history of sexual abuse. No erection or orgasm problems on either side. Latisha's low desire was specific to her relationship with Lucas.

Latisha was the oldest of three siblings. Her father left when she was 13 years old, and she never saw him again. She believed that he left her mother for another woman. Both of Latisha's brothers had been in trouble with the law most of their lives and her youngest brother was incarcerated at the time of treatment.

Growing up in a single-parent family allowed Latisha certain freedoms but carried responsibilities as well. Because her mother worked two jobs Latisha was charged with taking care of her younger brothers. And while this parentification (Boszormenyi-Nagy & Spark, 1973) came with certain privileges, she said that she felt tired most of her life. She not only had to get herself through school, but make sure her brothers were cared for. And because both boys were difficult, her job was that much more tiring.

While Latisha was a responsible person and a good student with college aspirations, she became pregnant by her boyfriend in her senior year of high school. Deciding to keep the child, a daughter, the couple moved in together right after graduating and formed a family. However, according to Latisha, after her daughter was born, the pressure was too much for her boyfriend and like her father, he left. Latisha was used to this lifestyle and just as her mother did, she worked two jobs to support her daughter.

Latisha reported that while her mother was a strong woman, she also seemed worn out by her responsibilities. She claimed that her mother was depressed and did not see a way out of the life she had found herself in. She also said that her mother gave her the message to be "independent" and to never get herself into the kind of situation she was in. She specifically warned her about getting pregnant and was terribly upset with what she called Latisha's "carelessness." She said that since Latisha got herself into this mess – meaning pregnant – she was not going to help her. She told Latisha that she was on her own.

While Latisha worked hard and never gave up hope of improving her life, she also demonstrated a tendency to sabotage herself. For example, after her boyfriend left, Latisha dated a series of men, all of whom proved to be irresponsible and selfish. When she finally decided to stop dating, a friend introduced her to a wealthy divorcee, Lucas. Latisha thought he was handsome and caring, and most of all responsible.

Lucas was the oldest child of three siblings. He was raised in a middle-class family in which college was a requirement, not a mere expectation. Both of his parents were college educated and his father was an accountant. He described his parents as ambitious but frustrated. He claimed that once he graduated law school and secured his first job, they began to expect that he would take care of them even though they did not have major financial problems.

Lucas claimed that although his siblings expected him to help them pay their day-to-day bills, his parents demanded that he buy them luxury items such as expensive cars or a vacation home. Lucas reported that he loved his parents and siblings, but he was often mad at them as well. Latisha validated this, noting that Lucas would sometimes snap at his parents and lecture his siblings when they would put pressure on him to help them.

Lucas was attracted to Latisha not only because of her physical attractiveness and her youth, but because she was an independent and hardworking woman as well. He was sure that she would not be too demanding of him and that she would be a great mother to his children from his first marriage. He really looked forward to marrying Latisha given his first wife became addicted to pain medication and unable to help him parent their two children. Like Latisha, however, he too had a series of post-divorce relationships with women who he believed were just after him for his money. He claimed they never had any intention of being a good stepmother to his children.

Interactional Style

This was a symmetrical couple with a confrontational–confrontational style. Latisha made it clear that she expected Lucas to meet her needs and to take an equitable role in helping her to raise her daughter. Lucas let it be known that he disliked being burdened and expected Latisha to carry out what he perceived to be her "wifely" duties of showing him affection and having sex with him.

Assessment Results

Latisha got the message from her beleaguered mother to make something of herself rather than rely on a man to support her. But her mother also told her to be realistic about her expectations in life. Her mother had experienced a lot of racism and sexism and gave Latisha the impression that being a Black woman would hold her back no matter how hard she worked. Latisha's mother conveyed unrealistically low expectations. This mixed message was in part responsible for Latisha's conflict around expectations. Being abandoned by her adulterous father and rejected by most of the men she dated were also contributing factors in making Latisha question her value. These messages and experiences help to create questions in Latisha's mind such as: What is the definition of success? How ambitious should I try to be? What is my worth? Do I deserve to meet my expectations?

Latisha did seem to expect a lot from herself; she wanted to live a better life than her mother had. But I believe that because of her conflict around expectations, she threw a few major roadblocks in her way to unconsciously sabotage this goal. First, she became pregnant young and ended up a struggling single mother. And like her mother, she was abandoned by her baby's father. Second, the men she chose to date were all similar: irresponsible and rejecting. And third, she married a man, Lucas, who had the means to help her achieve her goals, but he was conflicted about caretaking. And while Lucas was not an irresponsible man like many of Latisha's ex-boyfriends, he was like them in that he failed to meet her needs in the way and to the degree that she anticipated. She demonstrated unrealistically high expectations given the man she had chosen.

Lucas was trained to be a caretaker in his family of origin. The message he received from his parents was "a good son takes care of his family first and foremost." And while Lucas did his best to meet his parents' expectations, he also felt taken advantage of by them. Lucas did not mind buying them food or helping them with their mortgage, but he felt they were greedy and had little regard for how he was feeling.

His parents' demands were mainly responsible for his conflict around expectations, which he transferred to his relationships, especially Latisha and her daughter. He expected too much from them given the situation they were in. He wanted Latisha's daughter to be almost perfect, and if she wasn't, he would berate her. He also set extremely strict limits and according to Latisha, filled her daughter with anxiety. Once Latisha stopped having sex with Lucas, he felt emasculated and became even more demanding and selfish. He came to see Latisha like everyone else in his past – as a taker. He demonstrated unrealistically high expectations.

Clinical Recommendations

Both Latisha and Lucas needed to recognize their individual conflicts around expectations, how they shared this conflict, and how its unbalance led to their relationship symptoms. Specifically, Latisha had to abandon her mother's fatalistic perspective and not fear allowing herself to have a better life. In this process, she would have to grieve for her mother's plight and to let go of it. Her mother made her own choices, and the best Latisha can do now is to learn from her mother's mistakes, not replicate them.

Latisha would also have to process her father's abandonment and to accept that it had nothing to do with her value as a person. It was a problem that he unfortunately passed onto her. If Latisha is not in conflict about her self-worth, she will make the right choices in life, instead of sentencing herself to a lifetime of abandonment, rejection, and unfulfilled expectations.

To balance his conflict with expectations, Lucas must come to realize that his sensitivity to feeling burdened originated with his parentification (Boszormenyi-Nagy & Spark, 1973) in his family of origin. And while it is fine to set limits, especially with those who are greedy or who truly take advantage of him, he would have to own his ability to say "no" rather than overreact. He must also come to value close family relationships over materialism and recognize that he will never have this closeness unless he learns to accept some burden. In this sense, some burdens are worth the trouble.

Assessing Olga and Simon (See Figure 5.2)

The Initial Contact

Olga, an attractive 36-year-old Russian-born woman made the initial contact for treatment but said that her husband, Simon, 39, an American-born company executive with family roots dating back to the Revolutionary War agreed to accompany her, albeit reluctantly. The couple had dated for one year and had been married for five. They had twin girl toddlers.

Olga's chief complaint was that Simon had stopped having sex with her and was increasingly distancing from her and the children. She said that he was out a lot, and she had no idea where he was at any given time. When pressed, Simon would tell Olga that he was no longer attracted to her and that he wanted a divorce. He claimed that she could have whatever she wanted if she agreed to end their marriage. Olga suspected that Simon was having an affair, but she had no way of proving this.

Olga admitted she was the more assertive partner. She said that after yelling at Simon to change, she switched tactics and began to beg him to stay; neither worked. Two major points of contention were that Olga wanted her husband to send her to college in the United States and to help bring her parents and sisters here to live. She said Simon earns a lot of money as a Senior Vice President of a pharmaceutical company and easily has the means to do this for her.

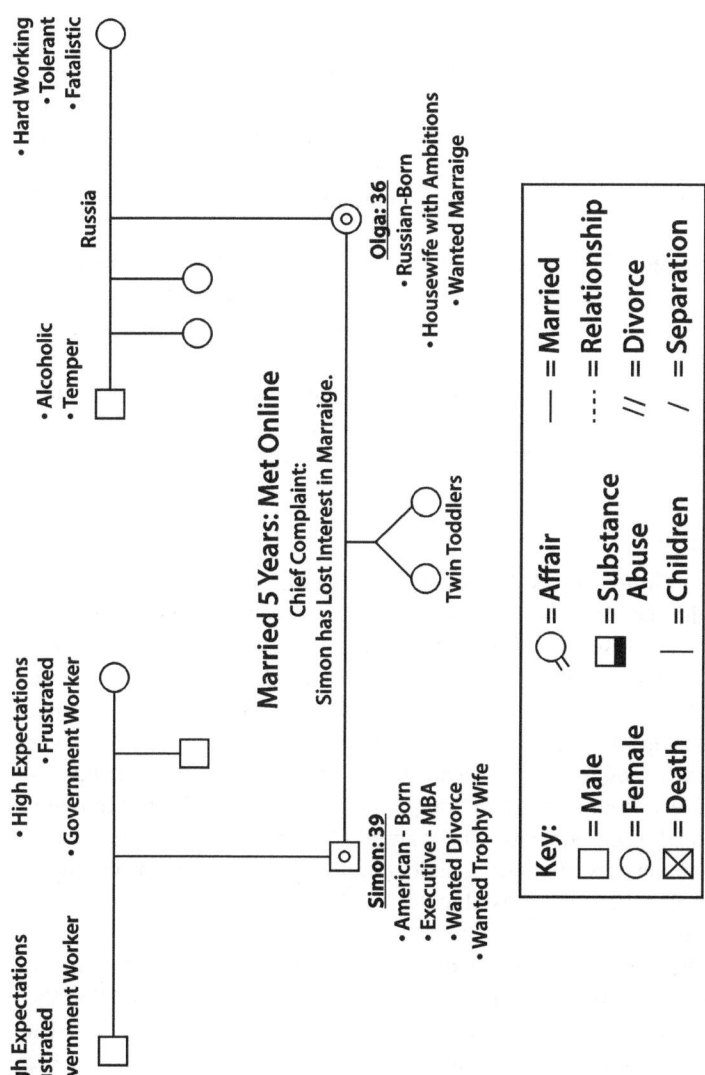

Figure 5.2 Olga and Simon.

The First Session

Simon said that he held no animosity towards Olga but that he could not give her what she wanted. He felt that he gave Olga a far better life than she had in Russia and that she should be grateful and take care of their two children. He said he never restricted her financially and if she left him alone and simply looked after the children, he would support them.

While Olga was not complaining about her lifestyle – she did appreciate all that Simon had been able to do for her and their children – she was vocal about expecting more of an equal relationship with him. She said that she feels as if she is a trophy wife for him to show off at his corporate parties. She came to believe that he had no intention of helping her grow as a person or helping her with her family.

Simon presented as a controlled, quiet man with little animosity towards Olga. He agreed to support her and the children financially and said that all he wanted was his freedom. He denied having an affair and claimed that he was not interested in meeting anyone else. He said that he needed a break and would not fight for child custody. Olga did not present as depressed, but she was befuddled by her situation. Indeed, Simon was elusive when it came to answering questions. He seemed like he was hiding something.

The Genogram

There was nothing remarkable about each partner's sexual history. Olga came from a traditional Russian family. She had two older, married sisters both of whom she was close to and who visited her in the United States every couple of years. She described her mother as an ordinary, hardworking woman and her father as a heavy drinker with an erratic temper. She said that her father could be embarrassing to the family when he drank too much and that her sisters and mother experienced the bulk of her father's drunken rage. While Olga's mother was a passive woman, she often complained to Olga that she felt trapped by her marriage to a "drunken fool." She warned Olga never to rely on a man for her survival, but she was also pessimistic about Olga's chances of making a better life for herself. The mother used to say to Olga that it was their family's fate to be miserable.

Despite her mother's mixed message, Olga had the courage to come to America with a couple of her Russian friends with the expectation that she could attend college in New York City and create a better life for herself. But soon after she got to New York she realized that could never afford to live there and go to school at the same time. She and her friends rented a small apartment, and she held two jobs. She eventually joined a dating website, and that is where she met Simon.

Olga said that she found Simon caring, handsome, and exciting. He also appeared confident, successful, and willing to start a family. While Olga preferred to go back to college with Simon's help, she acquiesced to his alternate expectation that she be a stay-at-home mother and raise their children. Olga was initially okay with this arrangement because she saw it as temporary. Once her children reached a certain age, she then expected Simon to help her gain an education even though he made no promises.

Olga and Simon had twin toddlers at the time of treatment, whom Olga thought were old enough to be looked after by a babysitter while she went back to school. But Simon disagreed and refused to pay for Olga's tuition. He said he was sticking to their original agreement.

Simon was the oldest of two brothers. Both of his parents worked for the United States Government, but they expected more from their children. Simon graduated from college and picked up a master's degree in business administration (MBA) later in his career. He eventually rose through the ranks of his company to senior executive status. He was well-liked and a team player. These attributes more than anything helped him to advance.

Simon reported his father and mother as similar in taste, values, and temperament. The only thing he could single out was that they were frustrated working for the government. Simon's father was especially sad and resentful that he had to leave college to take care of his sickly parents. On more than one occasion he told Simon that he had dreams of becoming a lawyer and that he regretted not having the chance. He warned Simon not to get himself trapped in a situation that would limit him.

Simon heeded his father's words, staying unencumbered by anything that would get in the way of his education and career, but he was admittedly lonely and longed for marriage and a family. When he was introduced to Olga, he saw her as smart, ambitious, and beautiful. But most important was that he saw her as a strong, independent woman who was sure of herself and quick to make decisions. And he was not wrong in his assessment of Olga. She came to the Unites States without knowing the language, found a place to live, and held down two jobs to support herself. This is hardly the work of a weak woman.

Interactional Style

Olga and Simon were a complementary couple with a confrontational–elusive style. Olga was the more confrontational partner. She asked a lot of questions, trying to better understand Simon's motivations for wanting to leave the marriage, but she got few answers. Simon was clearly ambivalent about treatment. He wanted to run away and hoped that Olga would let him go. Unlike other men he did not seem to care what the cost might be.

Assessment Results

Olga got the mixed message from her mother to be independent and not to rely on a man to support her. But she also conveyed a message that because she was from a poor family, it was her destiny to fail. I believe that her mother's message in part reflected a certain Russian fatalistic perspective. Her mother was a poor woman stuck with a mean, alcoholic husband in a communist country with no visible way out. No matter, I still saw this as unrealistically low expectations in relation to Olga. Yes, Olga was poor, but to be this fatalistic about her destiny was unrealistic, especially given Olga's drive and fortitude.

When they first met, Olga saw Simon as a sweet man who would not mind taking care of her and helping her gain her independence. He was fun and generous, and he was financially well off. Her conflict with her expectations, however, was primarily revealed in this choice of mate. She knew Simon was sensitive about anyone interfering with his desires and that she was to serve as his trophy wife. She was also aware that Simon's father warned him about not being tied down by anything or anyone, yet she married him and by doing so she demonstrated unrealistically high expectations for the marriage.

Simon did expect to care for Olga and their twin daughters to a certain extent, but his conflict revealed itself in his choice of a woman. That is, as much as he wanted to heed his father's warning to remain unincumbered, he longed for a family of his own and chose a woman who was strong and courageous but desperate and needy as well. His choice was indicative of his conflict with expectations – while he wanted a strong woman, by refusing to send her to college, he only increased her dependency on him. Simon demonstrated unrealistically high expectations in thinking Olga would settle for what he offered her.

Clinical Recommendations

Each partner must come to understand their internalized conflict with unmet expectations and to see how they share this with each other. Specifically, Olga did in fact want her dream of a better life fulfilled, but she needed to realize that she was working at cross purposes by choosing a man who was conflicted about responsibility. To balance her conflict and to better meet her expectations, she needed to see how her conflict was influenced by her family of origin. Specifically, she would have to move beyond her mother's fatalistic perspective, conquer the shame she felt coming from a poor, dysfunctional family, allow herself to feel more deserving of a better life, and to ultimately choose the appropriate male partner for the job.

To better balance Simon's conflict with unmet expectations, he would need to transcend his father's personal disappointments and separate them from his own fears. Specifically, Simon would have to balance his father's warnings about being burdened by the reality of what it takes to have his own, healthy family. He also needed to learn that it is acceptable to have needs and that he can meet his own needs and his mate's needs at the same time.

References

Aponte, H. (2017). Joining from the perspective of the use of self. In G. Weeks, S. Fife, & C. Peterson (Eds.), *Techniques for the couple therapist: Essential interventions from the experts* (pp. 11–18). Routledge.

Berman, E. (1982). The individual interview as a treatment technique in conjoint therapy. *American Journal of Family Therapy*, *10*, 27–37. doi: 10.1080/01921.188268250434

Betchen, S. (2005). *Intrusive partners-elusive mates: The pursuer-distancer dynamic in couples*. Routledge.

Betchen, S. (2022). *Couples in conflict: Clinical techniques for navigating sexual and relational control struggles*. Routledge.

Betchen, S. & Davidson, H. (2018). *Master conflict therapy: A new model for practicing couples and sex therapy*. Routledge.

Boszormenyi, N., & Spark, G. (1973). *Invisible loyalties*. Harper & Row.

Bowen, M. (1978). *Family therapy in clinical practice*. Aronson.

DeMaria, R., Weeks, G., & Twist, M. (2017). *Focused genograms: Intergenerational assessment of individuals, couples, and families* (2nd ed.). Routledge.

Doherty, W. J. (2002). How therapists harm marriages and what we can do about it. *Journal of Couple & Relationship Therapy*, *1*, 1–17. https://dx.org/10.1300/J398v01n02_01

Fogarty, T. (1979). The distancer and the pursuer. *The Family*, *7*, 11–16.

Gambescia, N., Weeks, G., & Hertlein, K. (2021). The sexual genogram in assessment. In K. Hertlein, G. Weeks, & K. Hertlein. (Eds.), *A clinician's guide to systemic sex therapy* (3rd ed.). Routledge.

Gottman, J, & Gottman, J. (2022). Enhanced Gottman Relationship Checkup. www.com/professioanls/gottman-relationship-checkup/

Hof, L., & Berman, E. (1986). The sexual genogram. *The Journal of Marital & Family Therapy*, *12*, 39–47. doi: 10.1111/j.1752-0606.1986.tb00637.x.

Lederer, W. J., & Jackson, D. D. (1968). *The mirages of marriage*. Norton.

Treadway, D. (2020). *Treating couples well: A practical guide to collaborative couple therapy*. Routledge.

Wachtel, E. (2017). *The heart of couple therapy*. Guilford.

Weeks, G., & Fife, S. (2014). *Couples in treatment: Techniques and approaches for effective practice* (3rd ed.). Routledge.

Section III

Clinical Treatment

6 Treating Couples with Unmet Expectations

Once the formal assessment phase has been completed and the couples therapist has gathered enough data to support a preliminary hypothesis that the couple is suffering from an unbalanced conflict with expectations, a general framework from which to treat has been set.

Treatment Objectives and Therapeutic Goal

There are several treatment objectives in MCT which are aimed at the goal of rebalancing a couple's shared conflict with unmet expectations and any associated nonsexual and sexual symptoms. To complete the objectives each partner must: 1) recognize that they have an internalized conflict with having their expectations met; 2) admit that they unconsciously strive to maintain this conflict to avoid the pain that usually accompanies change; 3) recognize the relationship between their unbalanced conflict and their symptoms; 4) recognize the pervasiveness of the conflict and how it might apply to other contexts or symptoms in their lives; 5) determine the origin of their conflicts; and 6) differentiate from their respective families of origin.

I employ a five-step process employed to meet these objectives and achieve this goal:

Step 1. Determining the couple's expectations and their connection to the couple's symptoms;
Step 2. Exposing the couple's conflict with having these expectations met;
Step 3. Broadening the context of the couple's conflict with expectations;
Step 4. Determining the origin of the couple's conflict with expectations; and
Step 5. Differentiating from the family of origin to better integrate and balance the couple's conflict.

Sometimes the steps overlap but once the last step is completed the couple is expected to be free of symptoms. The time it takes to complete each step depends on the intensity of the couple's conflict, the defensive mechanisms used to maintain the conflict's imbalance, and the couple's dedication to the overall therapeutic process. Several diverse cases will be used to illustrate these steps,

DOI: 10.4324/9781003359470-9

but because MCT includes the treatment of sexual problems, a brief section on sex therapy exercises will precede the case presentations.

Sex Therapy Exercises

According to Maximets (2022), when most people marry, they intend to satisfy, sometimes unconsciously, a wide array of needs and sex is one of them. Ballard (2021) reported that 1 in 10 Americans (10%) think it is fine to have sex within one week of starting to date, while approximately 2 in 10 (19%) believe it is optimal to wait one week or more but less than one month. Although this number is dependent on age, the average adult has sex 54 times per year (Twenge et al., 2017).

Research has indicated that sex is a vital component in relationships which can provide both mental and physical benefits (Brody, 2010). In a study based on 3,800 Chinese, sex was linked to overall happiness (Cheng & Smyth, 2015). And Monsesi et al. (2010) found that communicating about sex was important to a couple's overall relationship satisfaction.

Given these findings, it is no wonder when couples present for treatment with a sexual symptom they are distressed and wish to alleviate it as soon as possible. Many of the women that I have treated were angry about their partner's sexual difficulty, as if they were entitled to having a good sex life; an expectation many would not debate. Others, however, felt that their partner was no longer attractive to them or that they did something to cause sexual distress. Some think their partner had found someone better. A large-scale survey conducted in the United Kingdom found that 42% of the 1,000 women questioned about their partner's ED blamed themselves (Superdrug Online Doctor, 2022).

Nevertheless, because the MCT model is a psychoanalytic, psychodynamic approach, exercises are not "immediately" offered to a couple even if they present with a sexual symptom. And when they are prescribed, it should only be after a thorough evaluation of the couple's sexual history – including each partner's past individual experiences – has been taken and the shared conflict identified (see Chapter 5, Assessing Couples with Unmet Expectations).

Without knowledge of the conflict, it will be that much harder to suggest appropriate exercises and decrease the odds that any assigned homework will be successful. Even the most benign exercises like Sensate Focus I and II (Masters & Johnson, 1966) which are still useful (Avery-Clark & Weiner, 2018; Weiner & Avery-Clark, 2014)) could easily fail when an out-of-balance conflict with expectations is operating in the couple's collective unconscious.

Accordingly, the MCT therapist should refuse to assign exercises when deemed inappropriate. Rather, the therapist needs to skillfully weave together the couple's process or interactional style (e.g., Bickering–Elusive), their underlying conflict with expectations (e.g., having expectations met vs. not having expectations met), and their sexual content or sexual symptom (e.g., male hypoactive sexual desire disorder – MHSDD) with any potentially appropriate exercises. In previous writings I have referred to this as distinguishing content from process (Betchen, 2022, Betchen & Davidson, 2018). The following is an example:

Regina reported that her husband Saul had no sexual interest in her. After reading several articles on low libido she suspected that Saul had MHSDD, dragged him into therapy and immediately demanded sex therapy exercises. She said that she had been living with Saul's problem for the past two years and she has had enough. She also informed me that she fired the last three therapists they had seen because she was told that they had relationship problems not sexual issues. All three had recommended that the couple deal with their relationship first and that Saul's sexual desire would return.

The therapists were right in theory. But because they neglected to pay appropriate homage to Regina's desires, they were dismissed. A more productive way to approach this dilemma would have been to consistently keep the husband's low sexual libido in the therapeutic conversation while simultaneously addressing the couple's interactional style and underlying conflict with expectations. Consider the following example:

Therapist: Regina, I can see where exercises may be helpful in your situation. Judging from your history, you did not get a lot of your needs met as a child and Saul's sexual issue might be another example of this.

Regina: I never thought of it that way, but Saul is not even trying to fix his problem. He could live like this forever, but I can't.

Therapist: I can see it is a painful place for you to be. I sense that it sometimes causes you such anxiety that you cannot stop yourself from going after Saul. And when he runs from you, I suspect that increases your pain and lack of control.

Regina: (Quietly sobbing)

Therapist: Saul, was there a time when you enjoyed sex with Regina?

Saul: Yes of course. But I have not enjoyed much of anything for a while.

Therapist: Are you saying that you have not only lost your lust for Regina, but life as well?

Saul: I guess. I do not feel like doing anything.

Regina: Saul doesn't even have that much energy for the kids. I think he's depressed.

Therapist: Okay, when did you lose your mojo for life, Saul?

Saul: I think it was a gradual thing. But I don't think I ever recovered from being fired from the last job.

Therapist: How did Regina handle that?

Saul: She blamed me. She used to be very understanding but she changed. And I don't believe in divorce, so I've been feeling trapped. I can't talk to her because I am always to blame.

Regina: If the shoe fits...

Therapist: You expected more from Regina?

Saul: When I first met her, she seemed like a compassionate person. But I now think she's empathic to everyone but me.

Regina: I don't blame him for having a problem. But ask him what he has done about it. He hasn't even seen a urologist.

Therapist: You both sound disappointed in each other. I do think the previous therapists were right to suggest that there are relationship issues to be sorted out, but while we do that, how about trying a sexual exercise we call in the business, Sensate Focus I?

Regina: Finally, that's what we have been waiting for.

Therapist: I think you mean that's what you've been waiting for.

In this brief exchange. both content and process, and the conflict with expectations are given equal weight. This way, everyone's needs are met in treatment including the therapist who has escaped a double bind (i.e., premature termination by an angry couple or failed therapy courtesy of an inappropriate intervention). I was first taught how to elude a double bind in sex therapy by H. S. Kaplan (personal communication, October 7, 1987) who suggested that if a couple insist on exercises, the therapist might consider assigning Sensate Focus homework. Kaplan claimed that if these exercises failed, they were benign enough not to cause much of a therapeutic setback for the couple.

The Sabotaging of Sex Therapy Exercises

In MCT, the therapist should always remember that failure partially protects the conflict and so it is always looming particularly after a modicum of success. Because in the context of this book, a conflict with expectations is believed to underlie all sexual symptoms, the couples therapist should be prepared for each partner to take turns sabotaging the exercises, or for the couple to team up against the therapist to do so. This way the couple's expectations are not met.

Aside from pressuring the therapist to assign exercises prematurely, symptomatic partners may flatly refuse to do assigned exercises, or they may passive-aggressively sabotage them. The following is an example of a passive-aggressive man, Jack, struggling with his delayed ejaculation:

Linda: I had to drag Jack to treatment. He developed this problem soon after we moved in together and although he keeps telling me he will do something about it, he never does.

Jack: That's not true. I have made doctor's appointments.

Linda: Yes, but you cancel them or forget to go. It's even unfair to the doctors.

Jack: Something important always comes up.

Linda: Yes, obviously something more important than our sex life.

Jack had a history of not getting his needs met and of failing others, beginning with his hypercritical father. However, given his obvious resistance and Linda's insistence on exercises, I cautiously assigned Sensate Focus I.

Therapist: So, how did the exercise go?

Linda: Ask Jack.

Therapist: What about it, Jack?

Jack: I just did not have the time to get to them.

Linda: Yes, you did. You would rather play computer games than help us. I am not sure I can take this anymore.

Therapist: Jack, you say you are attracted to Linda and would like to fix your sex life with her, but I suspect that something is blocking you from giving it your all.

Other partners may move exercises along too quickly. Let's look at an example of this in the context of a case of Genito-pelvic pain/penetration disorder (GPPPD):

Tim: I think we are ready to go with the dilaters. I've been reading about them, and it seems they really work. I'm almost 40 and I want to have kids before it gets too late.

Dorothy: You're always pressuring me to do something, but I don't think I'm ready to shove these plastic-looking things inside me.

Tim: You've had a few years to do something about this and I'm tired of waiting.

Therapist: Tim, I know you're anxious and I see why, but if your wife isn't ready for this it may not work, and you will be that much more annoyed. I think it would be better to slow down a bit.

Tim: No way. I've waited long enough. She can try it or let's forget the whole thing.

Although the therapist tried his best to hold off Tim, Dorothy caved and tried the exercise. Even with the help of a lubricant, however, she was tighter than ever and unable to penetrate with the smallest of dilaters.

Jeremy and Sandy were inconsistent in treating the same disorder. This couple have been struggling to be consistent with the dilater exercises but instead took turns sabotaging them:

Therapist: Okay, how did the dilater exercise go?

Jeremy: Sandy tried it once but started an argument with me right before we were to do the exercise. I can't even tell you what she was upset about. She makes things up.

Sandy: That's not true. I asked you to take care of the dishes before I got home from work and you didn't, so I didn't feel like doing the exercise with you.

Therapist: It seems as if you two are conflicted about these exercises and improving your sex life. Prior to this incident the last time you tried the exercise was three weeks ago even though you are supposed to do them at least twice a week. It seems as if you take turns sabotaging them.

And last, some couples sabotage their sex therapy exercises by one or both partners taking control of them and changing what the therapists initially prescribed. The following example is that of Perry and Sue. This couple was struggling with Sue's female orgasmic disorder (FOD) or anorgasmia.

Therapist: How did the exercise go?

Sue: Not so good. Perry changed the rules.

Perry: I did not. You changed the rules.

Therapist: What do you both mean?

Sue: Perry was supposed to allow me to tell him when he could put his hand on mine while I was masturbating myself, but instead he grabbed me first. He also insisted that we do the exercise when the kids were home and we agreed in here only to do it when they were out so I would feel more comfortable.

Perry: First, I didn't "grab you." Second, the kids were in the basement playing. And third, you keep changing what the therapist says. You never give me the go-ahead to put my hand on top of yours.

Therapist: It sounds as if neither of you followed my recommendations. We should talk about this.

Selected Sexual Disorders and Exercises

As mentioned, MCT is not dependent on exercises in its treatment protocol, but sex therapy exercises have been found useful in treating a select number of sexual disorders listed below. Before reading on, however, please note that the MCT approach is not averse to incorporating medication in its treatment process. In fact, all those who present with sex disorders must have obtained a medical evaluation from a gynecologist or urologist before or soon after attending couple's work. It is also important to note that although the examples presented in this section are of straight couples, the exercises can be easily applied to gay couples as well.

Female Orgasmic Disorder

"Female orgasmic disorder (FOD) is defined as the absence, delay, infrequency, or marked diminishment in intensity of orgasm in at least 75% of sexual experiences, persisting for at least 6 months and causing distress…" (Marchand, 2021, p. 194). According to the *DSM-5*, the disorder "is not better explained by a nonsexual mental disorder or as a consequence of severe relationship distress or other significant stressors and is not attributable to the effects of a substance/medication or another medical condition" (p. 430). The disorder also consists of various subtypes: lifelong or acquired, and generalized or situational (American Psychiatric Association, 2013).

Approximately 40% of women have difficulty reaching orgasm and 10% never reach one with intercourse (Herbenick et al., 2018; Kontula & Miettinen, 2016). Stuparu (2020) claimed that FOD or anorgasmia is often presented in sex therapy. The treatment objectives being to improve communication, resolve conflicts, and cultivate self-exploration to alleviate fears, among others.

Freud (1905/1953) did a lot to set the table for female orgasmic expectations. In his clitoral/transfer theory he stated that women who could not achieve coital orgasm were immature and neurotic. He wrote:

> When erotogenic susceptibility to stimulation has been successfully transferred by a woman from the clitoris to the vaginal orifice, it implies that she has adopted a new leading zone for the purposes of her later sexuality. A man, on the other hand, retains his leading zone unchanged from childhood. The fact that women change their leading erotogenic zone in this way, together with the wave of repression at puberty, which as it were, puts aside their childish masculinity, are the chief determinants of the greater proneness of women to neurosis and especially to hysteria. These determinants, therefore, are intimately related to the essence of femininity.
>
> (p. 221)

If Freud did not give women enough reason to strive for vaginal orgasms, psychoanalyst Helene Deutsch was even more emphatic in her belief of the importance of the transfer in puberty from clitoral to vaginal sexuality. Deutsch insisted that that only vaginal sensations in response to the penis constitute normal mature sexuality, and that real sexual pleasure comes from the process of reproduction (Roazen, 2018).

Sexologists, beginning with Kinsey et al. (1953), have long rebuked the psychoanalytic belief that there were two types of female orgasm. Prominent sex therapists Masters and Johnson (1970) and Helen Singer Kaplan (1974) followed suit as do most sexologists today. Regardless, old prejudices are hard to ignore, and some couples still present for treatment with the belief that there is something wrong if the female partner cannot not achieve a vaginal orgasm. Some of the male partners report feeling emasculated and inadequate and some woman report feeling less of a woman and guilty for not performing. I find this even when the woman's clitoral orgasms are strong and satisfying.

In treating FOD, desensitization in conjunction with the psychodynamic work of uncovering the couple's conflict and connecting to the FOD is employed. Many women describe their anorgasmia as a "wall" that suddenly comes down and blocks them just before they are about to orgasm. Some have said that they often felt as if they were about to get there only to be disappointed and frustrated at the last moment. Still other women never get that close to orgasm and many avoid sex altogether for fear of stirring up something in them or their partner.

If a female client can achieve orgasm via solo masturbation, I usually skip individual exercises and proceed to work with the couple. If not, I will start by recommending that the female partner take time to be with herself, relax, think sexual thoughts, and stimulate her clitoris. I do not initially recommend the use of a vibrator for fear it can become addictive, but I will if all else fails.

Although the MCT model does not emphasize bibliotherapy, there are some women who are not very familiar with their bodies and have no idea what pleasures them; others are afraid to touch themselves. Many of these women are blocked by certain stereotypes and negative messages that counter their ability to enjoy sex to its fullest. In these cases, I might recommend books such as *Come as You Are* (Nagoski, 2021), *Becoming Cliterate* (Mintz, 2018) and for men *She Comes First* (Kerner, 2009).

Once the female partner can reach orgasm on her own, I move her to couple's exercises. Here there is a slow progression towards orgasm with her partner. I consider a clitoral orgasm a success, but if the couple, especially the woman wants to achieve a vaginal orgasm I will help them.

Exercises begin where the couple is currently; I have treated woman who can only achieve orgasm on their own *via* digital stimulation using their fingers, or with the use of a vibrator. If the woman is used to a vibrator and the couple wish to use it in their pursuit of orgasm, that may be an acceptable first step.

Other women cannot be anywhere near a man if they are to achieve orgasm and so I use the desensitization process to gradually bring the partners together. For example, one woman laid in bed masturbating to orgasm while her husband moved progressively closer to the bed with each session, until he was able to place his hand on hers while she used a vibrator to orgasm. The end of the treatment came when the woman achieved orgasm while her husband was inside her while stimulating her clitoris with a vibrator. That is all the couple wanted to achieve and so we all agreed to declare success. This case will be presented in greater detail later in the book.

Genito-Pelvic Pain/Penetration Disorder (GPPPD)

Sex therapy exercises are also used in the MCT model to treat a recently renamed sexual disorder now referred to in the *DSM-5* as Genio-pelvic pain/penetration disorder (GPPPD) (APA, 2013). This new definition combines the once separated dyspareunia or recurrent or persistent genital pain with intercourse, and vaginismus or recurrent or persistent involuntary spasm of the outer third of the vagina, hindering intercourse (Fertel et al., 2020).

The *DSM-5* suggests that for a diagnosis of GPPPD, symptoms need to be present for at least six months and cause significant clinical distress. Like FOD, the symptoms cannot be better explained by a nonsexual mental disorder or relationship distress. The disorder can be lifelong (i.e., no experience with pain free intercourse) or acquired (i.e., after a period of pain free intercourse) and rated from mild to severe (APA, 2013).

The exact prevalence of GPPPD is unknown and thought to be different depending on the age of the woman. For example, the estimates range from 6.5% to 45% in older women and 14% to 34% in younger women (van Lankveld et al., 2010). Rates also differ from country to country. The rate of GPPPD in North America was estimated to be 15% (APA, 2013) while a review of the literature on GPPPD in Spain found rates to be 11.23% (Berenguer-Soler et al., 2022). A study in Iran found rates to be 10.5% (Alizadeh et al., 2019) and a study in Australia found them to range from 3–18% (Bond et al., 2015). Rates have been reported higher in countries where marriages are arranged, polygamy is sanctioned, and widow inheritance are common (Amidu et al., 2010; Ysan et al., 2009).

The *DSM-5* has both dyspareunia and vaginismus listed under the more general category of pain disorder. But some studies still differentiate between the two in their research (Borg et al., 2011). I usually see women after they have been evaluated by their physician. Once the doctor determines that emotions are playing a part in their symptoms, even if an organic problem is present, I will treat the couple.

Couples expect to have sex when they form a union and to have children soon thereafter. GPPPD can prevent both expectations from being fulfilled. Because the MCT model integrates couples and sex therapy, it is most common for me to see couples with vaginismus who are either being threatened with divorce by the non-symptomatic partner because of a lack of sex, or because the threatening partner wants children and time is running out. Addar (2004) found that in 63.9% of cases, vaginismus was the primary reason for a couple's unconsummated marriage.

Integrating dilater treatment with the MCT approach has been successful in alleviating GPPPD, especially vaginismus. For example, a 38-year-old virgin conquered her vaginismus in time to enjoy sex and have children. But even though couples are often under stress to make progress, the woman should not be rushed through this process or it could backfire on the couple. This is especially true if the woman has a history of sexual abuse in which she was forced to perform sexual activities against her will. Rather, under the MCT model she moves at her own pace, while the therapist helps her to control her anxiety and block the couple's conflict from sabotaging the dilater exercises.

The woman can choose to insert the dilaters (preferably with a water-based lubricant) or have her partner do it. Regardless, they are to be used progressively (i.e., small to large) until the woman feels that her muscles are pliable enough and her anxiety level is such that she is ready to attempt intercourse. But this is easier said than done because if the couple's conflict with expectations is not under control, then the therapist can expect one or both partners to sabotage dilater treatment. For example, as I have written before (Betchen, 2010), when the non-symptomatic partner is about to get his needs met, he can sabotage the exercises. I tend to see this when the woman has one dilater left to complete the exercise. That is, he sabotages treatment just before the couple will be able to attempt intercourse. If the woman is going to sabotage the treatment, it is usually earlier in the process, or she might fail to make the transition from the fourth and last dilater to the penis. In some cases, anti-anxiety medication can aid the dilater process.

Premature Ejaculation (PE)

PE or "early ejaculation" is the most common male sexual disorder with rates ranging from 20–30% (Raveendran & Agarwal, 2021). The International Society of Sexual Medicine (ISSM) PE Guidelines Committee found the rates of acquired and lifelong PE much lower than most of the literature: approximately 4% of the general population. Nevertheless, because fewer than 10% of PE sufferers seek help it is difficult to get an accurate picture of the prevalence of the disorder (ISSM, 2015).

Men who have sex with men (MSM) refers to sex between men, no matter how they identify. Being a gay man is broader than being MSM; it is viewed as cultural identity (Mercer et al., 2016). Recent studies have shown the rates of PE for MSM to be lower than the rates for gay men (Barbonetti et al., 2019). But those MSM with PE, gay or otherwise, also suffer similar rates of distress as do straight men with the disorder (McNabney et al., 2022).

The *DSM-5* defines PE as "a persistent or recurrent pattern of ejaculation occurring during partnered sexual activity within approximately 1 minute following vaginal penetration and before the individual wants it" (APA, 2013, p. 443). To be considered a sexual disorder it should be present for at least 6 months and occur 75–100% of the time. It must cause significant distress and not be better explained by a nonsexual mental disorder or relationship distress. Like the other sexual disorders, PE can be lifelong or acquired, generalized and situational, and rated from mild to severe (APA, 2013).

PE is a sexual disorder especially susceptible to conflicts with expectations. Men with the disorder tend to blame themselves for their perceived inadequacy (Rowland et al., 2016). They also report more frequent sexual problems associated with increased anxiety and interpersonal difficulties (Fiala et al., 2021). Men with PE also tend to take responsibility for disappointing their respective partners (Rowland & Kolba, 2018).

Research shows that women in a relationship with premature ejaculators are disappointed with a truncated sexual experience, but this is especially true of women who can have vaginal orgasms. Partnered with a man who has PE makes many women feel as if they have been robbed of their own orgasm. According to Verze et al. (2018) these women also report sexual anxiety, poor sexual quality, and significant distress. They also experience greater stress being with someone who has this disorder and have attributed it to relationship breakups (Burri et al., 2014).

Traditionally the stop-start exercise (Semans, 1956) adopted by Kaplan (1974) and more modern sex therapists (Betchen & Gambescia, 2020) is now preferred over the squeeze technique (Masters & Johnson, 1970). The objective of the stop-start technique is to help the man with PE to learn to identify the pre-monitory feelings just prior to the inevitability of ejaculation.

The stop-start technique consists of the man stroking himself until he locates the point of ejaculatory inevitability and stops until the need to ejaculate is alleviated. He then begins to stroke again before he loses his erection. The man is to repeat this exercise several times until he feels confident that he is in control of his ejaculatory response. He can begin with a dry hand and then progress to using a water-based lubricant to better simulate the feel of a vagina.

Once the man successfully completes individual exercises, conjoint exercises are assigned if he has a willing partner. If the partner refuses, which is not uncommon, the partner is enabling the PE and likely has a conflict getting her needs met, which should be addressed. Some men can control the ejaculation process during masturbation. If this is the case, the therapist can bypass individual exercises and proceed to partner exercises.

Partner exercises consist of the female mate stroking the male partner until he identifies the point just before he will ejaculate so that she can stop stroking him. She may either hold the penis so it does not turn flaccid or let it go completely; this will depend on the man's sensitivity. She may first use a dry hand and then progress to using a lubricant.

While the female partner may sit near her partner when performing these exercises, the objective would be for her to place the man's penis progressively closer to her vagina until she is on top of him in the female superior position while stroking him. If all goes well it is recommended that once erect from stroking, she may insert her partner's penis into her and remain still for a few minutes not to trigger a quick ejaculation. This is a modified version of Hartman and Fithian's (1972) "quiet vagina" technique.

If the exercises do not seem to be working, the next step is for the man to try using a condom. And if this also fails, he might consider consulting a physician about taking a selective serotonin reuptake inhibitor (SSRI) such as paroxetine hydrochloride (Paxil) which are known to be used off-label to delay ejaculation. Waldinger (2013) claimed that an adequate ejaculation delay occurs in approximately 70–80% of PE sufferers within 1 to 3 weeks of initiating Paxil treatment.

Some men with both PE and ED may substitute the SSRI for a phosphodiesterase-5 inhibitor (PDE5) such as sildenafil (Viagra). Although originally developed to treat ED, these drugs also have been found to treat PE (Asimakopoulos et al., 2012; Gök-e et al., 2010; Hellstrom, 2010).

It should be made clear to the couple, however, that any medication suggested and prescribed will depend on a physician's examination of the symptomatic partner. The couples therapist should not have the final word on this subject. It is the physician's job when prescribing a medication to consider the individual's medical history and current medical status, and if there might be any potential negative side effects of the medication. Any potential for allergic reactions and deleterious drug interactions should also be held into account.

Clinical Case Examples

Having addressed sexual exercises, I will now demonstrate each of the MCT treatment steps using four clinical cases, two with nonsexual symptoms and two with sexual symptoms. Notice how the couples therapist consistently attempts to weave together the couple's symptoms with each partner's family of origin, their interactional style as a couple, and their shared conflict with expectations, to balance the conflict and alleviate their symptoms.

Krish and Amita: Nonsexual Symptom – Lack of Ambition (See Figure 6.1)

Initial Contact

Krish called to make an appointment for him and his wife Amita. This Hindu couple were in their late 20s and their three-year marriage was arranged in India. Krish came to the United States as a single, young man bent on securing a prestigious college degree in engineering. He did so and returned to India to marry Amita, who he had known since childhood. The couple then returned to the United States to seek their fortune. Amita attended college in India and worked as a laboratory tech once she was settled in the United States. The couple had no children.

Krish specifically called because he said that the marriage did not turn out like he expected. He said he thinks his wife has changed since coming to America. He said she is more assertive and independent; he expected her to remain passive and subservient. Amita has even threatened divorce, which was especially horrifying for Krish because he and Amita's families were close in India. Krish had known them his whole life. Krish said there is no indication that Amita was having an affair but that she has been very mean and distant to him for several months now.

Krish desperately wanted to save his marriage, but he said it is hard to make Amita happy and he's not sure what she expects of him. Kirsh said Amita agreed to attend sessions with him to make sure divorce was the right thing to do. He also said that he's sure that Amita also knew that her family would look down on a divorce and she is afraid of embarrassing them. Krish was hopeful but not optimistic about saving his marriage. He said he needed help. He told me that his wife was terribly angry, and he was not sure what she was so unhappy about.

First Session

Indeed, Amita was very angry, and it did not take long for her to say why she was considering a divorce. She said that Krish was lazy and that given how smart he

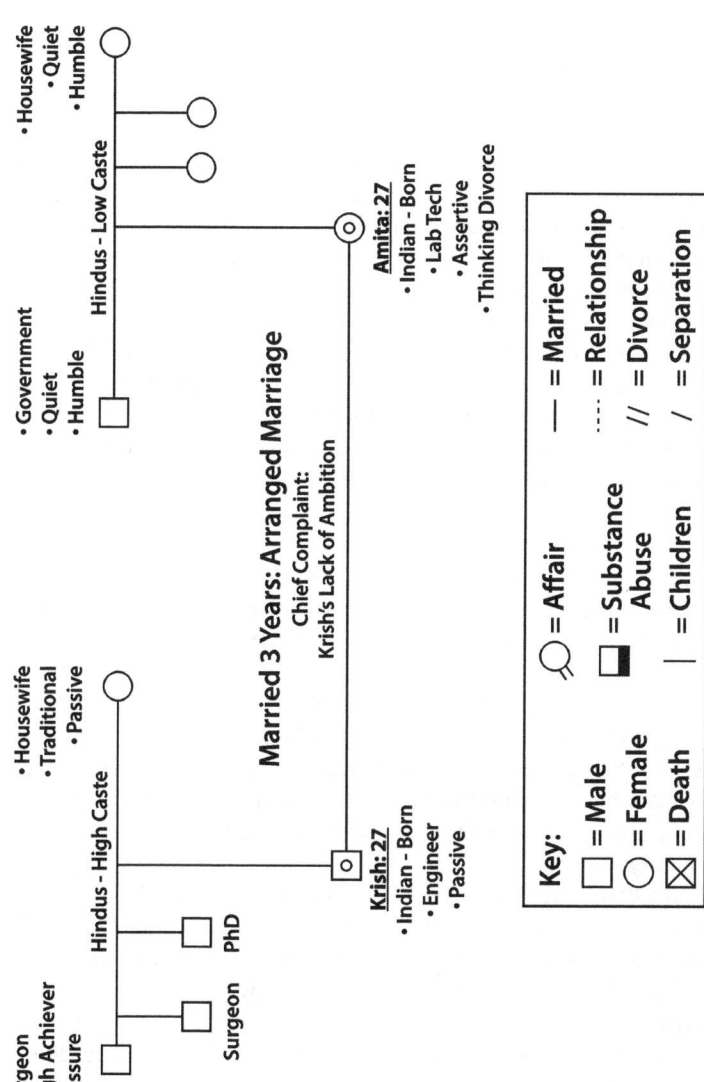

Figure 6.1   Krish and Amita.

is, he does not earn the money he could if he applied himself. She said that he is too meek to ask for raises. She also complained that Krish should also have obtained a graduate degree by now. Amita added that she no longer respects Krish as a man, and that she is not interested in having sex with him. She said that having children with him was also out of the question because she thought that the couple would struggle to support them.

Amita made it clear that she expected Krish to be more like his father and oldest brother, both prestigious surgeons in India. She did not think he would ever earn what a surgeon does. But she said this would not matter as much because they would be living a better lifestyle in America if Krish obtained a graduate degree and secured a job in a big company like IBM. Instead, Krish works for a small start-up company that is struggling to survive.

Krish said that he did not think he had the credentials to get into a large company and was ambivalent on whether to get an advanced degree. He was vague about this subject which made Amita even angrier. Krish did say that because both families were close and the marriage was arranged in India, he expected Amita to honor her oath and accept him as is. He added that money isn't everything and that it should not stop the couple from having children because his family was well off and eager to help. Amita said she would find taking money from his family embarrassing.

Genogram

Krish was from a higher caste in India than Amita. His father was an ambitious surgeon who always stressed excellence in education and his mother was a housewife from a very wealthy family. Krish described both parents as very demanding. They expected perfection from themselves and their children. Krish added that his parents did not take criticism well and were strict with him and his brothers. He claimed that there was little affection in his family; for that he relied on his maternal grandmother. He also claimed that status was particularly important to his parents and that they did what they could to always appear like the perfect family.

Krish was the youngest of three brothers. The oldest was also a successful surgeon and the younger brother held a PhD in Physics. Despite their achievements, however, Krish was considered the most intellectually gifted of the three children, having scored perfectly on his SATs, and getting into a prestigious college at an unusually early age. Surprisingly, however, he struggled in college, in part because he was very lonely and unhappy. He also said that college felt like a lot of pressure, and he had little fun because he had to focus on grades. He was happy to return to India to marry Amita.

Amita was the oldest of three sisters. She came from a lower caste in India, but Krish's father did not think that Krish deserved better because he did not do that well in college and rejected the idea of graduate school. He believed that only Krish's two brothers deserved women from higher castes and so he agreed to Krish's marriage to Amita. Amita claimed that this was the way it was in India, but she did hold this against his father.

Amita's father worked for the government and her mother was a stay-at-home parent. Neither of her parents were college-educated and she described both as quiet and humble. Amita said they were happy about their daughter's marrying into a higher caste.

Interactional Style

Krish and Amita presented as a complementary, confrontational–elusive couple. Amita was confrontational, which was unusual for a Hindu woman from a patriarchal society. Nevertheless, Amita did most of the talking and much of it was angry and threatening. Krish was meek and quiet, not the typical Hindu man. He would defend himself but in a way that was elusive and confusing. For example, while Amita was direct, Krish was vague. He certainly did not have a clear explanation for his lack of ambition or why he did not ask for raises at work or try to better his position with a graduate degree. And while Amita had higher expectations of Krish than he had of her, Krish did expect Amita to go against her nature and be satisfied with whatever he could provide for her. Given who Amita was, it could be said that Krish's expectations of her were grand, but in a different context.

Assessment

Although Krish claimed that he did not know what Amita expected of him, she was clear. Amita expected Krish to be a success in life. Specifically, she expected him to be a strong male figure with a successful career whose income was comparable to his father and brothers. Given his high caste in India and the success of his family members, she did not think that she was overestimating her husband's ability. But eventually she saw him as a lazy failure who disappointed her and disgraced both families. She felt he could do much better in life if he cared and he took more responsibility for himself rather than depending on his family.

Amita was not alone in her high expectations of Krish. His parents, especially his father, thought Krish should have surpassed all family members in career prospects and success. Krish let them all down according to his father. But given there was no indication – other than his intelligence and lineage – that Krish was ambitious and driven enough to achieve greatness – Amita and Krish's family demonstrated unrealistically high expectations for Krish. In fact, Krish had no interest in meeting their standards and made an argument to the contrary.

Amita's parents were average people from a low caste in India. And although they were pleased with Amita's ambitious nature, they seemed to have realistically low expectations for themselves that Amita refused to inherit. Although she loved them, she was embarrassed by their position and passivity, and strived to improve her lifestyle. This was at the crux of her conflict with expectations, and it showed.

Although an excellent college student majoring in biology in India, rather than pursue her dream of medical school she decided that it would be too much work and took a job in a lab. And while life has been easier academically, she has never forgiven herself for not pursuing her dream. She also felt inferior to Krish and his family, despite Krish's failings. Her conflict was also evident in the way in which she handled Krish. Rather than uplift him and offer positive reinforcement, she chose to denigrate him, which only served to increase his passive aggressiveness and his sense of inferiority.

Krish demonstrated a conflict with expectations in that he came from a family that had it all, but he chose not to use their resources to better himself. There were no mixed messages from his parents. They were traditional Hindus who believed in a patriarchal system with the man as the breadwinner. In fact, Krish's family was even willing to send him to graduate school, but he procrastinated, making excuse after excuse. It was as if he was reluctant to meet his family's expectations of him and by doing so, he turned his wife into an angry parental figure.

As mentioned, Krish expected Amita to settle for what he could provide for her given her lower caste. He worked hard enough to get by and did not have to worry about money because he knew that his family would help financially in a pinch. He saw Amita as disloyal and greedy. His perception of her threat to divorce was viewed as a breach of her marital oath to him and to their respective families. He took no responsibility for angering her. He demonstrated unrealistically high expectations in thinking that Amita would settle for what he offered.

Amita's parents agreed that their daughter should live a better life. They too were relying on Krish to make this happen. The only difference between Kris's parents and Amita's parents were that the latter were humble, poor, and less confident. They seemed honored that Amita was accepted into a family from a higher caste.

The sexual assessment of the couple was unremarkable. Both partners were virgins when they married and claimed to enjoy sex early in their marriage. Once it became apparent that neither were going to fulfill each other's expectations their sex life deteriorated. This took about two years, but it was not until then that Amita decided she was no longer physically attracted to Krish. Krish felt differently. He continued to want to have sex with Amita and was sad when she refused. Amita also chose to withhold affection from Krish and with that the couple grew more distant.

There was no history of abuse of any kind reported and no paraphilias or fetishes. Neither partner was on medication although Krish was experiencing some anxiety and having difficulty sleeping. Given these symptoms, he was considering talking to his physician about a trial of anti-anxiety medication.

Treatment

Step 1. Determining the couple's expectations and their connection to the couple's symptoms.

It was easy for the therapist in this case to make the connection between the couple's conflict and their symptoms given what was revealed in the assessment. But getting the couple to see this is another issue. Partners are usually well-defended, and in this case, neither was too eager to take any individual responsibility for their part in the marital breakdown. The following is a brief exchange demonstrating how the therapist helped this couple to make this connection:

Therapist: Amita, I get the sense that marrying Krish was not what you expected.

Amita: No, Krish had all the things he needed to become a success. But instead, he squanders these things and doesn't try to make our lives better.

Therapist: What things are you referring to?

Amita: His parents are rich. He went to the best schools, and he is very smart. He is just lazy.

Therapist: So, you thought when you were matched up with Krish that he had a bright future?

Amita: Of course.

Therapist: You sound angry.

Amita: I am.

Therapist: Angry enough to withhold sex and to threaten divorce?

Amita: I cannot live like this.

Therapist: You also sound as if you're in pain.

Amita: (Crying) Yes, and he will not do anything about it. I'd rather leave than put up with this.

Therapist: You did not have the advantages that Krish had, did you?

Amita: No. But if I did, I would show some respect.

Therapist: If you did you would expect more from yourself.

Amita: Yes. I would not let everyone around me down and disgrace those who have given so much to me.

Therapist: You're awfully quiet, Krish.

Krish: Yes.

Therapist: Any thoughts?

Krish: I just do not think I'm as bad as Amita makes me seem. And my family is not disgraced by me.

Amita: They do not say much but I can tell they are.

Therapist: You think Amita is being unfair in her characterization of you?

Krish: I am not as driven as she wants me to be, but I make a decent living. We do not need fancy cars or a huge house.

Amita: You are just making excuses for your laziness.

Therapist: Krish, is what Amita is saying shocking to you?

Krish: Well, I just do not think I'm as big a failure as she is making me out to be.

Therapist: So, you think she's being unfair?

Krish: Yes.

Therapist: And is that what you expected from Amita?

Krish: No. I expected her to stand by me. Not to put me down all the time. And even if I am not a surgeon, she has more with me than she had with her parents. It all makes me want to do even less. What is the point?

Therapist: So, you both have let each other down.

Step 2. Exposing the couple's conflict with having their expectations met.

Therapist: Amita, did you see anything in Krish that might have given you a clue as to what his values were about work and money?

Amita: He graduated from the best schools.

Therapist: Yes, but did you know, for example, that he struggled in college and that he felt under a lot of pressure to succeed?

Amita: Yes. Krish told me about not liking it when we got together. He did say that a part of him wanted to quit but he knew his parents would disown him.

Therapist: Any other signs that he may not have been as ambitious as you say you would have liked?

Amita: Not that I remember.

Krish: I told her that all I want is for us to get married and settle down. That I did not need fancy things. I just wanted a small home and to start a family.

Therapist: Do you remember him telling you that Amita?

Amita: Yes. But I thought he would change his mind and want more. Everybody usually does.

Therapist: Apparently Krish is not one of those people. Amita, it sounds as if you had signs that, despite Krish's background, he was not ambitious and didn't particularly value it. But you ignored the signs and got yourself into a place with which you are unhappy. Now you are a smart woman, so I can't help but believe that you are in conflict about getting your expectations met or you would have paid more attention to the signs.

Krish: Yes, she knew what I was like.

Therapist: And I suspect you knew her as well. Krish, weren't there any clues that Amita wanted to move up in status and saw you as an avenue to do so? Weren't there any signs that she wanted more for her children than she had as a child?

Amita: Of course. I told him many times that I hoped that our children would have the privileged life he did. He knew I wanted them to go as far as they could in life.

Krish: Yes. She did tell me that.

Therapist: And yet you went through with the marriage knowing she was looking for more than you expected to give. I would have to say that this feels like a conflict about what you expected her to put up with.

Krish: Yes. I see that.

Step 3. Broadening the context of the couple's conflict with expectations.
To figure their problems out, many people focus on what is in front of them and miss the bigger picture. Unfortunately, this miscue often results in an unconscious replication of their problems. For example, because a middle-aged woman had been abused emotionally (e.g., name calling) and physically (e.g., punched and kicked) by her father and ex-husband, she swore that she would be sure to avoid this kind of man when dating. As soon as a man showed any semblance of temper, she immediately ended the relationship. However, what she failed to recognize was something much more general. While focusing on a man's overt temper she consciously chose a passive aggressive man. But even though they presented differently, the passive man also withheld his feelings and took advantage of her financially. He was also quite distant from her children.

To increase a couple's insight into their conflict with expectations, the couples therapist needs to find at least one other context in which each partner has experienced unmet expectations. This way, rather than blame each other for their individual unmet expectations, they will have to take individual responsibility for having a conflict with expectations independent of their partner. In the following example, notice that the therapist sometimes allows partners to answer for each other. This is one way the therapist can bypass any resistance from a partner who is asked a specific question. It also helps with forgetfulness.

Therapist: Amita, how does it make you feel to know that Krish is not reaching his potential as you define it?

Amita: I think he is being unappreciative.

Therapist: Yes, but what feelings do you get? I hear the anger and disgust in your voice but are there any other feelings?

Amita: I feel mostly disgust because I know what it is like to not have the advantages he has.

Therapist: In comparison to his upbringing, do you feel cheated?

Amita: Well, my parents did the best they could, but I always felt a little embarrassed and resentful as a child. But again, they did the best they could.

Therapist: So, that sounds like a conflict of sorts. And you have had this your whole life. Has anybody else ever made you feel this way?

Krish: She is upset with some of her friends who are wealthier and never offer to help her. And she has complained more about her parents than she is letting on. When she did not get into a prestigious college, she was mad at them. Anytime someone mentions college she gets upset.

Therapist: Yes, it sounds like this issue has been around.

Amita: Well, Krish is certainly not helping me with it.

Therapist: He might be exacerbating it, but it doesn't look like he is the cause of it. Krish, have you ever felt the feelings you now experience with Amita?

Amita: I can answer that. Krish is usually passed over for promotions at work, even by people less qualified. But he never fights for what he deserves.

Krish: It does not bother me as much.

Therapist: As much, or never?

Krish: Well, sometimes, but I don't obsess over it the way Amita does.

Therapist: When does it bother you?

Krish: I guess when my friends get raises and I know they are less skilled than I am.

Amita: Ask him about his brothers.

Therapist: Okay, what of them?

Krish: I get a little angry when they buy expensive things. And I hate it when they brag.

Amita: He also gets angry when he hears what athletes and celebrities make. Sometimes he yells at the television.

Therapist: Well, Krish, it sounds as if the issue that's bothering your wife, bothers you independent of her.

Step 4. Determining the origin of the couple's conflict with expectations.
Krish was no doubt under a lot of pressure from his parents and extended family to become successful. For example, his father saw him as the child with the most potential despite how accomplished his other sons were.

While Krish wanted to please his family and compete with his brothers, he simultaneously despised the pressure of competition. Because this conflict was out-of-control, Krish unconsciously chose to marry Amita, a woman from a lower caste. Amita was desperate to move up but because of her conflict with expectations, she was more critical than supportive of Krish, thereby ensuring that neither would get their expectations met.

Krish and Amita needed to see the connection between their shared conflict with expectations and their respective families of origin. The following is an example of how this was achieved in treatment:

Therapist: Krish your parents sounded as if they had faith in your abilities.

Krish: Yes. They expected more from me.

Therapist: But you have done well. You are an engineer.

Krish: Yes. But not a surgeon or a famous scientist. Engineers are respected in my culture but I'm an average engineer with an average income.

Therapist: We have established that a part of you wants to be more successful, but there is also a part of you that doesn't want the pressure.

Krish: I see that now. I did not before.

Therapist: Where do you think that comes from?

Krish: I know the part of me that wants to achieve comes from the pressure my parents put on me and my brothers. But I do not know where my resistance comes from.

Therapist: Well, how do you feel about the pressure?

Krish: Scared. It is too much for me. And having my brothers do better than me increases the pressure. I was supposed to be the star.

Therapist: Any other feelings?

Krish: I do not think so.

Therapist: How about anger?

Krish: What do you mean?

Therapist: Your parents set the bar for you. Some people would be upset with them for being so demanding.

Amita: You are angry Krish. But you are afraid to admit it. Instead, you curse your brothers. But they are only responding to the demands of your parents.

Krish: I never thought of that. But in my culture, it is disrespectful to argue with your parents.

Therapist: So, Amita is right?

Krish: Yes.

Therapist: Your conflict is connected to your upbringing in that part of you wants to please your parents and compete with your brothers, and the other part of you refuses to do so. This latter part of you is rebelling. In this way you make it difficult to meet your own personal expectations, but you anger and disappoint Amita and your parents.

Krish: I never thought of it like that. But Amita does act like them in how she treats me.

Therapist: Amita, you have admitted that you want Krish to be more successful, but do you really think you are helping him?

Amita: Nothing seems to work. As I have said before, he is lazy.

Therapist: I remember, but you have always wanted to move to a higher caste but I am not sure you're comfortable with this.

Amita: What do you mean?

Therapist: I mean that if you wanted to get your expectations met you would have bettered yourself rather than solely rely on Krish. You had a chance to be a doctor. You also might have found a way to support, rather than criticize him. This reflects a conflict with improving your place in life. Contrary to popular opinion, it is hard for people to improve their status. Some feel as if they are abandoning their family of origin; others feel like an unworthy imposter.

Amita: (Crying) I want a better life so bad. But sometimes I feel like it is my karma not to get it. I was born into this caste, and I cannot escape it. I love my parents but I am also angry with them for putting me in this situation.

Therapist: I think you can have a better life. But not without negotiating with your conflict.

Step 5. Differentiating from the family of origin to better integrate and balance the couple's conflict.

To rebalance his conflict, Krish needed to integrate the side of him that wants and expects to achieve and the side that wants to rebel. That is, he would have to find some compromise between the two sides. The first step would be for him to admit that his conflict has had a negative impact on his finances, self-esteem, and his marriage and that the price he pays to rebel is greater than the price to succeed. This is vital because people cannot change unless they see the value in the change. Change is just too hard without hope.

Krish would also have to curb his anger towards his parents, especially his father, and to set goals and work towards them. He would have to come to the realization that even if his father's pressure tactics left little to be desired, it does not mean that he was wrong about his son's talent and the virtues of achievement. While this may sound easy, for some just the thought of working harder might prove anxiety provoking or depressing. It changes the way one lives and requires greater effort and discipline. It also requires caring more and risking failure.

To balance her shared conflict with expectations Amita will have to grieve her position in Indian society. She will also have to give up her anger for her parents and her cultural system and to look to improve her position rather than rely on others like Krish. While Krish can help, Amita must battle her position by birth and reject its limitations. As Ross (1995) suggested, for some it is easier to move down than up.

The following is an example of how the therapist worked with Krish and Amita to help them to differentiate from their respective families of origin, alleviate their symptoms, and to balance their shared conflict with expectations:

Therapist: Krish I know that you do not want to lose Amita, you have said so. But I am not sure what you are willing to give up, to keep her.

Krish: I am not sure what you mean.

Therapist: You know what her expectations are so are you interested in meeting them or not?

Krish: Well, I think that her expectations are unrealistic.

Therapist: That is interesting because one side of each of you is in sync. That is, there is a part of you that wants to achieve more and to make those around you happy. This is what Amita wants for you.

Krish: Yes, but she wants too much from me.

Therapist: I am not so sure about that. The other side of her fights against meeting her own expectations.

Krish: I never looked at it that way.

Therapist: Yes. In some ways, she is just as blocked from meeting her own needs and yours as you are from meeting your needs and hers.

Amita: I see what he is saying, Krish. He is saying that I am conflicted about achieving and I am blaming you for my conflict. I am having trouble meeting my own expectations, so I want you to do it for me. That is why I am not helping either of us.

Therapist: Precisely.

Krish: But I do not agree with Amita's values or my parents.

Amita: Part of you does. I can no longer blame you or my parents for this. But you must do something as well to save us.

Krish: I do not understand.

Therapist: How would you feel if you started to work harder and to set and pursue goals?

Krish: I guess I would feel like I was giving in. Giving in to my father and to Amita.

Therapist: Yes. You would have to stop battling them. But before you can do so you must believe that to continue the battle could be detrimental to you and your sense of self, and fatal to your marriage.

Krish: I know what I am doing now does not seem to be working.

Therapist: Well, I am calling for a compromise of sorts. You do not have to win the Nobel Prize. But you do need to stop battling enough to see what you can accomplish. You can then see what you have to offer or what your true capabilities are. It will take courage, but I suspect your parents were not entirely wrong about you. They do have an eye for talent.

Krish: What about Amita?

Therapist: Amita must grieve her natural position in life and prove to be less conflicted about moving upward than she is. This way both of you can better meet all expectations, including those of both sets of parents. It is not perfect, but at least your conflict will be under control, and you will be fighting less.

Michael and Sharon: Nonsexual Symptom – Feeling Unloved (See Figure 6.2)

Initial Contact

Michael and Sharon were an interfaith couple (i.e., Jewish and Episcopalian) in their late 50s who had two grown sons. The couple had been married for 25 years. Michael, a successful car dealer, called for an appointment because he was caught having an affair. While his wife Sharon, a teacher, was not threatening divorce, she refused to speak with him after finding out about it and this was causing Michael a great deal of anxiety. Michael was scared primarily because he did not know how Sharon would respond. Would she cheat on him? Would she divorce him? Michael claimed that he wanted to save the marriage, but he saw himself to be at Sharon's mercy.

According to Michael, he and Sharon met at college the first year and dated on and off until the couple married soon after graduation. This was Michael's one and only affair and he claimed there was no emotional attachment involved. The woman worked for a competitor and Michael met her at a car auction. They were only together a handful of times, but the affair was exposed when Sharon noticed that the woman was trying to contact Michael on his cell phone.

First Session

In the first session, Sharon appeared angry. She raged about all the things Michael had done to her over the years. When she got to his affair, she repeatedly asked him why he did it. Michael said little but did express remorse and called himself an "idiot." When I asked if he knew why he had an affair he said that the couple have not had sex in two years, although he never addressed the issue with his

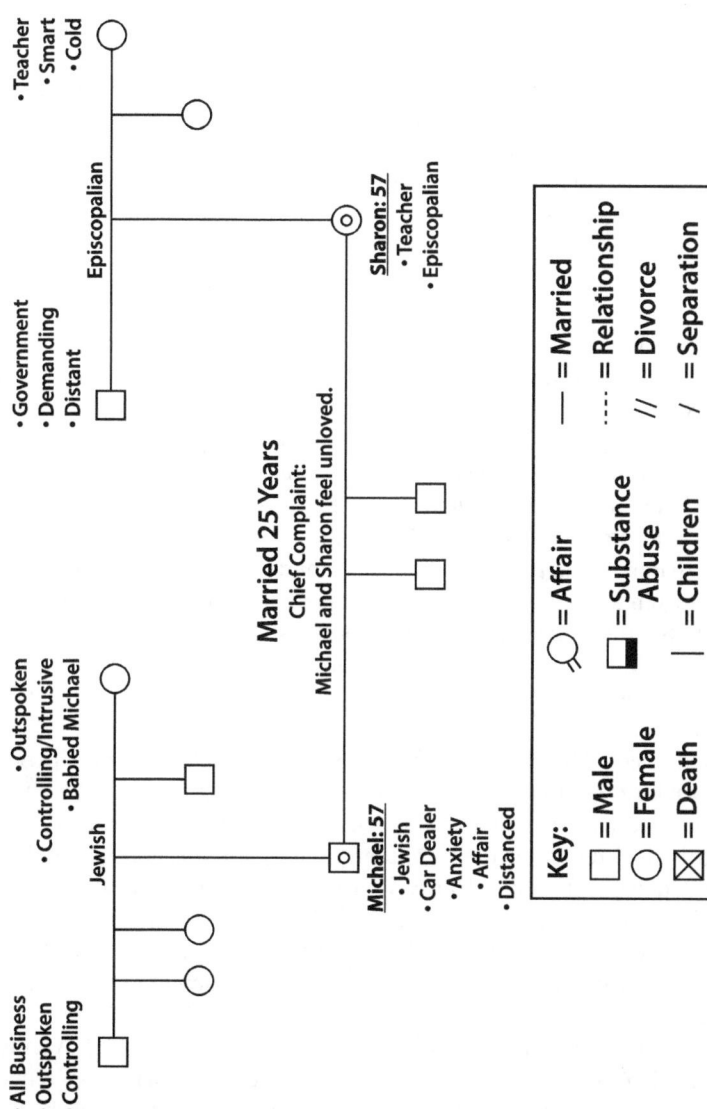

Figure 6.2   Michael and Sharon.

wife. When asked to comment, Sharon said that she had been living without sex as well but that she did not have an affair.

When the couple were questioned about their early dating, they admitted to having a strong sex life. Both were virgins when they met in college but did have a fling or two during some pre-marital intermittent separations. The couple also reported that when mad, Sharon would pursue Michael and Michael would distance *via* his work. This would make Sharon even angrier.

When asked what they expected from each other Sharon claimed that she wanted Michael to be monogamous and to make her a priority in his life. Michael claimed that he too wanted to be a priority to Sharon and that he expected her to have sex with him. Although they could express their expectations, neither was sure how to meet the other's needs.

Genogram

Michael comes from a conservative Jewish home. His parents were uneducated but started a family car dealership that is still remarkably successful. Michael is the only sibling in the business. He has two sisters and a brother. Michael admitted that he had a privileged upbringing but that his parents were very outspoken and controlling. He also said that his father was "all business." Michael said that he knew that his father loved him, because he rarely refused help but that he was not an emotional man. Michael claimed that his mother "babied" him.

Michael's parents disapproved of Michael's marriage to Sharon on the grounds that she was from a financially modest Episcopalian family. His mother simply did not think Sharon was good enough for him. Michael's family even refused to attend his wedding to Sharon, and since that day he and Sharon have had an estranged relationship with them. Michael claims that he only talks business with his father out of necessity.

Sharon felt rejected by Michael's family. She claimed that from the first time Michael introduced her to them she felt they were looking down on her and that it only got worse after they had married. She claimed that she believed Michael's family also looked down on their children as they are not considered Jewish because in Judaism religious identity is based on the mother, not the father. Sharon said she never felt accepted, and Michael treats her as a second-class citizen as well. Michael disagreed and told Sharon that he loved her and that he risked his family for her. He felt that should be worth something. Sharon just rolled her eyes.

Sharon came from a middle-class background. Her father was a government employee, and her mother was a schoolteacher. She claimed that her parents did not have difficulty accepting Michael but were justifiably worried that she might be rejected by his family. Sharon described her mother as smart but cold, and her father as very demanding and distant, especially when you failed to please him. Sharon has one younger sister who lives "far away."

Sharon said she never had high aspirations other than marrying and having a family. She was fine with Michael's ambitiousness, but she was not okay with him placing his work ahead of her or their children. Michael did not deny this and admitted there was a flaw in his character. He said that his parents taught him to work hard and to be successful and that is what he does. He said that he knows that Sharon expected to be the top priority in his life but that he is not sure how to do that. Michael expects Sharon to be happy with all he can provide for her and to have sex with him. But he also wants affection and feels that she is not in love with him and never has been.

Interactional Style

Michael and Sharon were a symmetrical, bickering–elusive couple. Sharon was angry about being treated unfairly by Michael and his family and would cite numerous incidents depicting these injustices. She claimed that she would beg Michael to spend more time with her, but he would disappear into his work. There were times that he would not return her cell phone calls for hours. Michael did not deny Sharon's many accusations but could not seem to explain his behavior other than he wanted to work. He did, however, blame his affair on the couple's lack of sex, but Sharon countered that if she felt loved, sex would not be a problem. Michael did not believe her but had no alternate explanation. Like Krish and Amita, both Michael and Sharon had grand expectations for one another. Michael wanted affection and sex from Sharon even though he did little to earn it; Sharon expected Michael to make her, not his work, a priority in his life even though he never has.

Assessment

Michael claimed that he was his parents' favorite, especially his mother's. He said that his mother indulged him and that he had to do little to please her. He even said that she could be delusional about his achievements in school and in sports, exaggerating them to others. Michael said that of all his siblings he got the best grades and went to an Ivy League college so there was some justification in his mother's belief in him. He also showed the best business acumen and even his father, who was less indulgent, thought he would be the one to take over the business and to take it to new heights. It was apparent that Michael's parents had realistically high expectations for Michael. Michael's conflict with expectations was evident in his expectation to be catered to, as he was in his family of origin, without earning it. This dynamic was evident in his marriage to Sharon. He wanted Sharon to show him affection and to have sex with him even though he routinely distanced from her and treated her like a second-class citizen.

Sharon described her home life as void of emotion. There was also little guidance or encouragement to succeed even when she showed some academic promise. It was as if she raised herself. Sharon claimed that her parents treated her much like Michael's parents did. It was evident that Sharon's parents had unrealistically low expectations for her. Her conflict, which she transferred to her marriage to Michael, was that she wanted to be loved but unconsciously was not sure she deserved this kind of attention. Both Michael and Sharon demonstrated unrealistic high expectations for each other given their relational interactions and their personal histories.

The couple's sexual history supported a conflict with expectations. For example, although they had satisfying sexual relations from the time they met in college and for the first few years of marriage, they did break up several times over the years and slept with other people. This demonstrated how little they valued each other. According to Michael, the couple would decide to resume their relationship because they could not find anyone better suited. That is, they each treated their relationship from the beginning as a business "transaction" with little love and affection for one another. Neither partner was ever a priority for the other, although they both claimed to expect this.

According to the assessment, neither partner was abused sexually. There was no evidence of porn use, fetishes, or paraphilias. Neither had an extensive sex life given they were both virgins when they met in college and spent much of their adult lives together. Any other sex came when the couple would periodically separate.

Treatment

Step 1. Determining the couple's expectations and their connection to the couple's symptoms.

Both Michael and Sharon were conveying the message that each expected to be treated as a priority. Specifically, Michael expected more affection from Sharon, and he expected her to have sex with him. Sharon expected Michael to show more interest in her, and to prioritize her ahead of his work. She also expected him to be faithful.

Both partners had great difficulty taking individual responsibility for their contributions to the symptoms. For example, Michael admitted the affair was wrong, but he could not see how his neglect of Sharon caused her to stop having sex with him. Sharon saw no excuse for Michael's affair whatsoever. Rather than focus solely on Michael's affair and enable the couple to continue to simplify their dynamic, I chose to open them up to expectations they were unaware of and connect these to their symptoms. I saw this as an easier way to reach them. The following is a brief example of how I achieved this:

Therapist: Michael, when did the sex stop?

Michael: A few years ago.

Therapist: Nothing since?

Michael: Nothing. I have tried a couple times over the years, but Sharon wasn't interested. So, I decided rather than push her, I'd try to focus on other things.

Therapist: Do you mean like an affair?

Michael: I know. That was a bad idea. But I needed sex, and I wasn't getting it at home.

Therapist: Are you suggesting that your affair is a direct result of not getting sex at home?

Michael: I think so.

Therapist: Really? I suspect it is more complicated than that. Is that all you expected from Sharon... sex?

Michael: I think so.

Therapist: Well, if that is true, why did you decide to have an affair now, after all this time of not having sex?

Michael: I have no idea. It just happened.

Therapist: If Sharon begins to have sex with you again, will everything then be fine?

Michael: No not really.

Therapist: Right. You expect more from her, so let us hear it.

Michael: I want Sharon to love me and show me affection.

Therapist: Is that it?

Michael: I want her to support me. I supported her when my parents rejected her.

Sharon: You did. But now you reject me.

Michael: What does that mean?

Sharon: Work is your priority. I was important to you.

Therapist: Sharon, is there a direct link between those feelings and the stoppage of sex?

Sharon: I think so.

Therapist: Right. Because you stopped the sex long before the affair.

Sharon: Yes.

Therapist: So, Sharon, what are you missing?

Sharon: I want to be loved as well. He defended me against his parents so why couldn't he keep making me feel special? What happened?

Therapist: Sharon, are you suggesting that you really stopped sex because you didn't feel loved?

Sharon: I can't sleep with someone who treats me like Michael does.

Michael: I don't know what happened to me. I guess I got caught up in my career.

Therapist: But Michael, you've been successful for a long time now. It can't just be work that's blocking you.

Michael: I don't know. But I do love Sharon.

Sharon: Really. You certainly fooled me.

Step 2. Exposing the couple's conflict with having their expectations met.

Exposing a couple's conflict with expectations in a way that they can process to their advantage is an arduous task. Often, this is where the couples therapist is faced with each partner's individual defenses and their defenses as a united front. The following excerpt demonstrates how to challenge these defenses to expose the conflict:

Therapist: Michael, I am a bit confused. You say that you have wanted to have sex with your wife for some time. You say that you love her and are still attracted to her. And yet you had an affair. I would think that this behavior would only make your chances of having sex with her even more remote.

Michael: I know. I said it was dumb.

Therapist: But you are not a dumb person. Have you told her how unhappy you have been?

Michael: I think so.

Therapist: You are not sure?

Michael: She knew.

Therapist: It doesn't sound as if you were that assertive about it. You also have admittedly not made her a priority in your life and have in fact spent most of your energy on your career. This makes some sense to me, but you continue to do so even though your car business is thriving and you have achieved great financial success.

Michael: Well, I didn't feel that important to her so I put my energy into something that I thought would have a better payoff.

Therapist: Yes, but you weren't really satisfied with that decision, or you wouldn't have felt the need to have an affair. It sounds as if you were trying to have your cake and eat it too. That is, you put your energy into work and found another woman to satisfy you. You wanted it both ways. And yet you said that you are more attracted to your wife than this other woman and that you love your wife.

Michael: Yeah, I know.

Therapist: So, do you or do not you want to have sex with your wife? Do you or don't you want to save your marriage?

Michael: Yes, to both.

Therapist: Are you sure? Because if you are, you will have to demonstrate it. Sharon does not seem to believe you. I'll put this in business terms: Your credit is questionable.

Sharon: That is a fact.

Therapist: Michael, I suspect that you have been sabotaging your expectations of Sharon.

Michael: I see what you are getting at. Whatever I say that I want, I do something to prevent getting it.

Therapist: Correct. But not consciously. You want Sharon to meet your needs and yet, you do something that will make it so she will not want to. It is as if you are trying to get what you want without earning it and it never works. And Sharon, I suspect you do the same.

Sharon: What do you mean?

Therapist: Now do not misunderstand me. I am giving Michael responsibility for the affair. But you say you want him to love you, but you vacillate between bickering at him and distancing yourself from him. You have put the kids ahead of him, and you spend more time with your friends. You also claim to want a monogamous relationship, but you have stopped having sex with Michael. How could you ever expect to get what you want out of this relationship with those tactics? This points to a conflict about getting your expectations met. I wonder if you are questioning whether you deserve to be loved.

Sharon: I do not know. But I see what you are saying.

Step 3. Broadening the context of the couple's conflict with expectations.

This couple's conflict with expectations was not confined to their relationship. For example, Michael expected his parents to accept Sharon, but they still do not. But he should have known better because his parents had made it clear that they wished their children to marry within their faith. It also did not help that Sharon was not from a family of means and Michael knew his parents were judgmental and materialistic. Hence, Michael knew how his parents might react but still chose to bring Sharon into his family. Michael's conflict also showed itself in his unrealistic high expectations of his business partners and employees. He often demanded more from them than their work ethics and talents allowed.

Sharon also knew what her future in-laws would be like, but she married into Michael's family where she was rejected and discriminated against. She also had some difficulty with her friends, expecting them to take her side against Michael while they tried to stay neutral. The following is an example of how the treatment helped the couple to expand their view of how their conflict functions in contexts other than their marriage:

Therapist: Michael, what expectations do you have for your children?

Sharon: None. He doesn't talk to them.

Michael: I talk to them. But I do not think I put pressure on them if that's what you are getting at. I expected them to finish college and the rest is up to them.

Therapist: How about you Sharon, what expectations do you have of them?

Sharon: Not much. I don't pressure them either. They are good kids.

Michael: How about your employees Michael, do you expect a lot from them?

Sharon: He is brutal to them and easily loses his temper.

Michael: Yeah, I'm not a great administrator and then I get mad at them for not being able to please me.

Therapist: I guess they must make a lot of mistakes. This reminds me of your relationship with Sharon. You expect your employees to meet your needs, but you set them up to fail. What about you Sharon, do you have friends?

Michael: Talk about expectations. Sharon expects everyone to agree with her or she will dump them. But what she asks of them is sometimes impossible.

Therapist: Like what?

Michael: I can't speak about her friends, although she is known for cutting people off if they don't agree with her. But with my parents she knows they are limited in what they will do for us and how they react. But she keeps expecting them to warm up to her. But they do not even warm up to me. I used to expect better behavior from them, but I now see that they cannot change. And they're older and even more stuck in their ways.

Sharon: He is right about his parents. I keep expecting them to accept me and they won't. I want to let go of that, but I think it's wrong of them.

Therapist: So, as individuals it can be said that you both have expectations of others, many of which are unrealistically high either by your hands or theirs. If this is true, you both brought this conflict to your relationship and you both have difficulty supporting one another.

Step 4. Determining the origin of the couple's conflict with expectations.
Although the partners were told that each of them brought their own internalized conflict with expectations to the relationship, it is easier for them to accept this if they can make the connection between their conflicts and their respective pasts. The following is an example of how this was achieved in treatment:

Therapist: Michael, did you see much affection growing up in your family?

Michael: Not between my parents, but my mother "babied" me. She loved me too much. But it did make me feel special.

Therapist: How about your father, did he show you affection?

Michael: No, he was not an emotional man.

Therapist: You said your mother loved you too much. What does that mean?

Michael: She was all over me.

Therapist: So, she took good care of you, but she was intrusive.

Michael: Yes, it was too much. I was her favorite. I couldn't do anything wrong, and it was easy to please her. She would do anything for me. And while this was good, it made my siblings upset and I needed more space.

Therapist: That sounds like a conflict in the making.

Michael: I never thought about it.

Therapist: You want to be treated as if you are special, but it costs you.

Michael: Yes. I see your point.

Therapist: It seems like that's what you want from Sharon.

Michael: I miss the sex.

Therapist: Well, yes. But what are you willing to put into it? You want what you want but you do not want to be tied down and earn it. It is the deal you had with your parents.

Michael: I see the connection.

Therapist: Sharon, you claim to expect more from Michael. Did you get your needs met in your family?

Sharon: I never thought that much about it.

Therapist: Now is a perfect time to try.

Sharon: My parents could be cold. I was on my own.

Therapist: So, you had to take care of yourself.

Sharon: For the most part. I mean they fed me and put a roof over me. They paid for college.

Therapist: Yes, but it does not sound as if your emotional needs were met.

Sharon: No.

Therapist: So, you then marry a man who had his own troubles getting his needs met, other than financially. And you expect him to help you. This might be evidence of your conflict: you miss getting your needs met, especially the emotional ones, but at the same time you are not used to it. All courtesy of your family of origin.

Step 5. Differentiating from the family of origin to better integrate and balance the couple's conflict.

This is the most challenging part of the therapeutic process and the time when a couple's defenses are most activated. It is the point in treatment when the couples therapist lets the couple know that to balance or rebalance their shared conflict with expectations, they will have to give up something deep within them; something beyond their awareness. This is the only way to alleviate their symptoms and there is no gain without pain and sacrifice. The following is an example of this process in couple's treatment:

Therapist: Sharon, you claim to want your emotional needs met and to be treated as a priority by Michael. I do think these are reasonable desires given Michael is in conflict. But I am not convinced as to whether you can tolerate having them met by him. That is, if Michael successfully grapples with his conflict, it might not be good enough. You may just raise the bar.

Sharon: You mean because it has taken so long. I do admit I am angry.

Therapist: No. What I mean is that because you too are not used to getting your needs met, how do we know that you will let yourself be satisfied?

Sharon: Do you mean because of the conflict?

Therapist: Yes. I suspect that somewhere inside you, you do not think you deserve to get your needs met. And, you will have to let go of the anger you have, not just for Michael, but for your parents as well. This might be the only way you can allow someone to please you. In other words, you will have to let go of the way you were treated as a child to balance your conflict with expectations and to allow others like Michael to meet your needs.

Sharon: But even if I can, Michael still might not give me what I want.

Therapist: True. But you will know what to do in that case because you won't be as conflicted about it. Michael must do his part. He must acknowledge that to meet both of your needs, he will have to risk putting more into his relationship with you and in a sense, earn your love. He must therefore give up his specialness and work for what he wants. He will both gain and lose something in this decision.

Michael: It does sound hard. Will this solve our issues?

Therapist: It will not make either one of you perfect. But there is no such thing as perfection, especially in us humans. Neither of you will ever feel completely whole because of the way you were raised. But if you better manage your conflict, you will evolve into a less transactional team. That is, control over your shared conflict with expectations should help each of you to get more of your needs met.

Dean and Maxine: Sexual Symptom – Genito-Pelvic Pain/Penetration Disorder (Vaginismus with Exercises) (See Figure 6.3)

Initial Contact

Maxine, a 34-year-old architect, called for her and her husband Dean, a 32-year-old government employee. Maxine said that they needed someone who could help with both couples and sexual problems. The couple had been married for five years and had no children. This was the first marriage for each partner. Maxine claimed that she was diagnosed with vaginismus by her OBGYN and

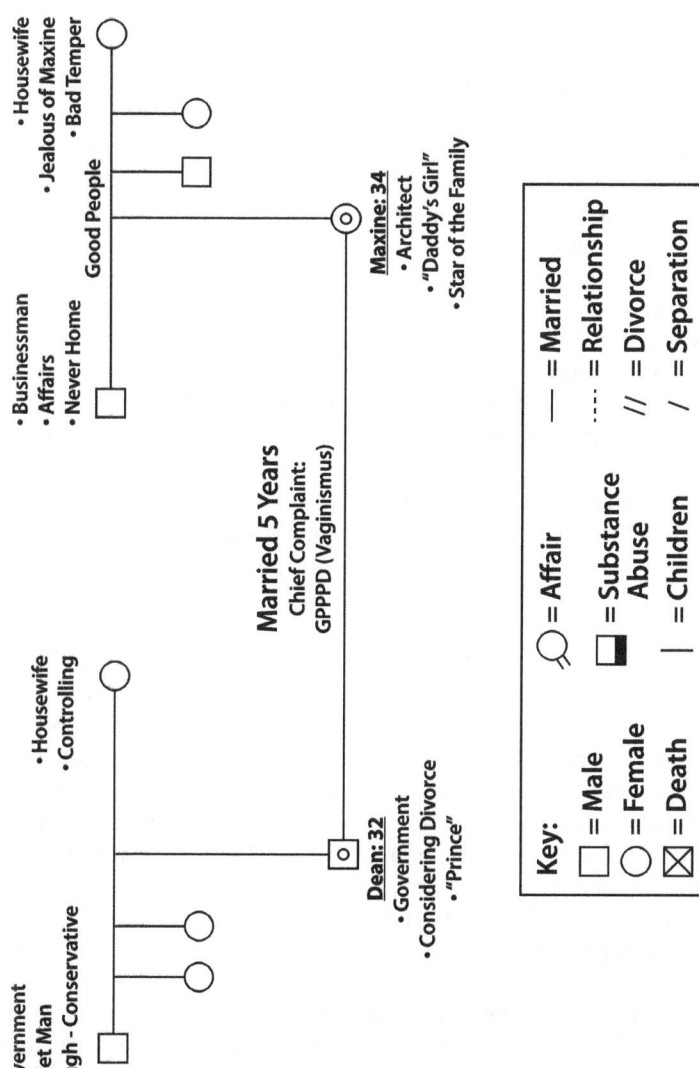

Figure 6.3   Dean and Maxine.

has been unable to have intercourse for the last two years. The couple used to engage in other forms of affection, including oral sex, but as their mutual anger and resentment grew about the vaginismus Maxine put a stop to all sexual intimacy. Maxine said that Dean is increasingly upset and considering divorce.

First Session

Maxine began by saying that she did not know what to do about her sexual problem. She said that she wished she could have sex with Dean because she still found him attractive, but intercourse was too painful, and lubricants did not help. Although she initially felt bad for Dean, she now feels angry and hurt. She said that she expected Dean to be more understanding but that he has been difficult from the beginning.

Dean was both annoyed and sad. He complained that when they dated, he and Maxine had great sex together, and that one of the main reasons he married her was because he found her extremely sexy and irresistible. He expected a great sex life with someone he found so attractive and was sad that she could no longer have intercourse with him especially without pain. Maxine intervened and said that she could not function sexually because of the pain but now she is also too angry anyway. She said that Dean expects her to just put this problem out of her mind and it will miraculously go away. She also said that Dean claims that she is using this problem to maintain sexual distance from him. She could not believe that Dean was being so unreasonable and unsympathetic.

Genogram

Maxine is the oldest of three siblings. She was an excellent student in high school and college and graduated from a top architecture school. In her junior year of college, Maxine was recruited by a large city architecture firm and quickly rose to partner status. At the time she met Dean, she was earning a hefty salary.

Maxine was the star of her family of origin and had the confidence and freedom to take risks. She left home immediately after high school and moved to Chicago to attend college. Maxine's siblings were not as daring and still live close to their parents. Her brother is a computer programmer in a small company and her sister is a paralegal. Both are married to what Maxine calls "average people."

Maxine described her parents as generally good people, but they had their problems. She said that her father was an astute businessperson with money, but he was never home. She said that she missed having him around because when he was present, he made her feel like "daddy's girl." Nevertheless, Maxine suspected that her father had many affairs, and this in part made her feel sorry for her mother, a housewife.

Dean was the youngest of three siblings and the only male. He admitted that he was treated like a "prince" growing up, not only by his parents but by his sisters as well. His father was described as a quiet man who, like Dean, worked for the government. But he was a tough, conservative guy who was often critical of the way his son was babied by other family members. His mother was said to be more of a force in the family who controlled the homelife with an iron fist.

Dean remained close to all his family members, especially his mother and sisters, and had a nice circle of friends. He had one relationship in his early years, and he reported no sexual difficulty. But the relationship did not last in part because his family did not approve of the girl. Maxine claimed that another reason it took Dean so long to settle was because he had to get final approval of any girl he considered from his mother and sisters. Maxine said they believed that: "No girl was good enough for their little Dean."

Interactional Style

Dean and Maxine were a symmetrical, confrontational–confrontational couple. Both partners were outgoing and talkative but still open to new information. While Maxine was slightly more assertive than Dean, he was not afraid to speak his mind or to fight back. At times, the couple could become loud and off point, but they responded well to the structure of the treatment when confronted.

Assessment

Maxine enjoyed being the star of her family, but she also felt guilty about her good looks and believed that her mother was jealous of her. Maxine's parents thought so highly of their daughter's beauty they were certain she was destined for stardom – perhaps an actress. They had realistically high expectations for Maxine. But Maxine was not without conflict. Although she loved being the star, she hated that her poor mother was jealous of her. She even attributed her mother's bad temper to her frustration with not being as pretty and popular as her.

Maxine also despised being made to feel like a sex symbol to men who did not see her as a serious mate. Maxine denied any sexual abuse, but she did say that she had to fight men off most of her life. She pointed out that architecture was a man's field, and that she had to deal with a lot of sexual harassment over the years. She also said that she was always aware of her good looks and her figure, and she knew that most men just wanted to have sex with her. She had many male encounters over the years, but most expected sex from her and were often relationship phobic. She said, "you would think that my looks would keep a guy, but they often worked against me." Maxine admitted that even though she knew the temporary nature of her relationships, she never experienced vaginismus with any man. Maxine's conflict around expectations showed itself in the shallow, narcissistic men she chose, and her vaginismus with Dean.

Dean enjoyed his princely status in his family of origin, but it came with a price: he had to find the perfect woman. This led Dean to be overly discriminating about who he would date, severely limiting his choice of women. He admitted that he feared bringing dates home because he did not want to subject them to his mother and sisters.

Dean grew to dislike the limitations that came with being a prince and he was concerned that his father was annoyed by it and saw Dean as less of a man. Unlike his wife and daughters, he did not think Dean was perfect or anything close to it. Dean's mother, on the other hand, had unrealistically high expectations of Dean. She did think he was perfect. Dean also longed for marriage and a family but had to wait until he found the perfect woman for fear his mother and sisters would criticize him and that he would let them down. Dean admitted that Maxine was not perfect, but he knew that his family could not deny her beauty and personality.

It was clear that Dean and Maxine shared a conflict around expectations, even though both claimed to want to have their expectations fulfilled. Dean wanted affection and sex from his wife but the way in which he treated her all but guaranteed he would not be successful. In fact, his entitled attitude made matters worse. This behavior was consistent with Dean's family of origin: He was treated like a prince and expected his needs to be met.

Dean stated that he expected sex from Maxine and that he felt betrayed by her. He saw her as a very sexy woman and took it personally that of all her lovers, she shut down sexually on him. This, according to Dean, has impacted his sense of masculinity. Dean vacillated between anger and sadness about his situation and was threatening to divorce even though he said that he did not want to take this route. It was clear that he was still attracted to his wife.

Despite his expectations, Dean's conflict was evident by his inability or refusal to empathize with his wife and to help her with her vaginismus. Instead, he was critical and demanding, which only made her more upset with him. In time, his reactive style only served to erode whatever affection and sexual play that existed. He persisted with unrealistically high expectations for Maxine.

Maxine wanted to keep her marriage. But she was upset with Dean's impatience and lack of empathy. He was the love of her life and she expected more of a commitment from him regardless of the problem. She said that she would do what it would take to rid herself of her vaginismus but beyond seeing her OBGYN, her conflict revealed itself in that she procrastinated in seeking sex therapy for two years. She admitted that Dean was always demanding when it came to sex, but that he was far less patient with her now. Her avoidance led Dean to replace whatever empathy he did show with anger. Maxine likewise had unrealistically high expectations of Dean.

The assessment did not reveal abuse of any kind in either partner's pasts. Maxine had many successful sexual experiences, far more than Dean, and had no other sexual issues. She could freely masturbate to orgasm and when feeling healthy could achieve a vaginal orgasm with intercourse.

No paraphilias or fetishes were evident and both partners claimed to remain very attracted to each other. Neither partner took medication, but Maxine was considering something because of the pressure from Dean and the stress of the overall situation.

As mentioned earlier in this chapter, vaginismus is one of the sexual disorders determined to be a common symptom in couples who have a conflict with expectations. Having sex is thought by most couples to be a given, especially in long-term relationships or marriage. When it is perceived as being withheld, no matter what the reason, it often causes great turmoil for the couple. To treat this specific disorder, sex therapy exercises in the form of dilater treatment is employed along with the couple's psychotherapy.

Treatment

Step 1. Determining the couple's expectations and their connection to the couple's symptoms.

The expectations of each partner were obvious. Dean wanted Maxine to show more affection and to have sex with him. He knew that intercourse was painful for her, but he was frustrated with her and demanded a solution. He was especially upset that she procrastinated in seeking treatment for her problem.

Maxine expected empathy from Dean. She believed that if he loved her, he would be more patient with her and help her to get over her problem. As mentioned, both claimed to still be attracted to each other. The following exchange shows how the couple's expectations were linked to their sexual symptoms:

Therapist: Dean, you seem to believe that Maxine is intentionally withholding sex from you.

Dean: I don't know. But I used to be more understanding. Now I'm tired of not having a sex life. Maxine could have dealt with this issue sooner.

Therapist: I am only asking because you seem to be upset with her, not so much the problem.

Dean: Well, I do think she procrastinated.

Therapist: Do you know why she did that?

Dean: No.

Therapist: You do not seem to care about what the reason is.

Dean: At this point I don't care. A wife is supposed to have sex with her husband. I am supposed to do certain things as a husband, and she is supposed to do certain things as a wife. And I am not even sure what vaginismus is.

Therapist: Did you go with her to the doctor?

Dean: No.

Therapist: Okay. So, you are upset with Maxine because you expect her to do certain things that she is not doing, namely, have sex with you? And if she were able to you would be fine?

Dean: Yes. Well, I might still be a little upset for this taking so long. But I would feel better than I do now. I know it can be painful, but she didn't even seem interested in even using a lubricant.

Therapist: Maxine, why did you procrastinate getting treatment?

Maxine: I think I was scared. And I thought Dean would understand that.

Therapist: Did you tell him you were scared?

Maxine: Yes. But he didn't seem to care. He thinks he was patient and empathic at first, but he really wasn't. He was better than he is now, but he pressured me and made me feel that I was not fulfilling my end of the marriage contract from the beginning.

Therapist: How did you feel about that?

Maxine: First I felt guilty that I had this problem. But then I got angry.

Therapist: Because you thought it was Dean's job to be more empathic?

Maxine: Yes. I see what you are trying to say. That we had certain expectations and instead of dealing with them the right way we made things worse.

Therapist: Something like that. I suspect he made you feel like your old boyfriends did: like a body for service.

Maxine: Yes. That's it!

Dean: But I am not an old boyfriend.

Therapist: Right Dean. And you expected to be treated as if you were special.

Step 2. Exposing the couple's conflict with having their expectations met.

As mentioned, both Dean and Maxine acted and reacted in ways that ran counter to having their expectations met. The following exchange shows the couple how this reflects their conflict with expectations and how this conflict is responsible for their sexual problem:

Therapist: Dean, you say that you want Maxine to show you more affection and to have sex with you, but it seems as if you have no clue how to make this all happen.

Dean: Like I said, I used to be understanding but she has pushed me to the limit.

Therapist: Well, according to Maxine you were annoyed from the beginning; you were just a bit more in control.

Dean: That is her perspective. I thought I was very understanding. But when it was clear that she was procrastinating I could no longer control my anger.

Therapist: Okay. So, you admit that you were angry from the beginning, but you were able to control it. Is it not possible that some of the anger showed itself... a little bit?

Maxine: Come on Dean, tell the truth.

Dean: Maybe.

Therapist: I would think so. Look Dean, I'm not blaming you for wanting to have sex with your wife. But instead of supporting her, you made things worse. Now how could that help you to get your needs met?

Dean: I don't know.

Therapist: When I usually see a person who is working at cross purposes it makes me think that person is conflicted about what they say they want.

Dean: But I really don't think it would matter. I think nothing will change Maxine.

Therapist: I won't debate that with you because you may, in fact, be right. But you need to leave that up to Maxine. At least she would not be able to sit here and blame you for her problem. Maxine, you say you want more empathy from Dean, but you procrastinated in seeking treatment and you stopped whatever sexual activities you were having. It is as if you severed whatever ties you had to your husband. That too is not making things better. In fact, it is evidence of the same conflict Dean has. How can you expect more empathy from Dean if you continue to annoy him?

Maxine: I see. So, you are saying my behavior is evidence that I have a conflict with my needs as well.

Therapist: Yes.

Step 3. Broadening the context of the couple's conflict with expectations.

At this stage in the process, the therapist helps each partner to see that their conflict with expectations is not limited to their relationship. Rather, the conflict exists in other contexts of their lives as well.

Therapist: Maxine, are there any other areas of your life that cause you difficulty?

Maxine: Like what?

Therapist: Like work?

Dean: Tell him about your ongoing problems with the head of the firm, Maxine.

Maxine: Oh, it's no big deal.

Dean: Yeah [sarcastically]. No big deal, it just costs her raises.

Therapist: Maxine?

Maxine: Okay. He thinks I do not get enough of my projects done on time. It's not the quality of the work, but he does think I focus too much on detail and miss a lot of deadlines.

Therapist: And has this cost you?

Maxine: I have been passed over for some rate increases.

Therapist: You mean he has not told you what he expects of you?

Maxine: He has.

Therapist: So, as with Dean you expect to be rewarded by not doing what he wants?

Maxine: Well... when you put it that way...

Dean: What about you Dean? Does your conflict apply to other areas of your life?

Dean: I don't see it.

Maxine: Come on Dean. Dean feels as if the world owes him. He fights with his parents and his friends when they do not give him what he wants.

Therapist: Yes. But is what he wants doable?

Maxine: Normally it would be, but who he expects it from does not make any sense. And he ends up disappointed. For example, he expected that a colleague of his would confess that Dean would be better promoted to a management position but instead his friend touted himself for the job. Dean felt really betrayed but the world does not work that way. Dean now hates the guy and won't even look him in the eye.

Maxine: You also expect your parents and sisters to put your needs above their own. And although they try you get mad whenever they cannot.

Dean: Yeah. I guess I am a bit spoiled.

Therapist: That is why you had difficulty with Maxine not meeting your needs. But you just did not handle it in a way that would help you get what you say you want. The main point here is that your conflict also operates in other contexts.

Step 4. Determining the origin of the couple's conflict with expectations.
There was no apparent trauma or incident, past or present, that might have contributed to Maxine's vaginismus. But it was evident that her husband's sexual expectations conflicted with her high expectations of him which in turn, caused her to withdraw. But there were deeper reasons for the behavior of both partners in this dynamic and to get to these reasons each partner would have to connect their current behavior to their pasts.

Based on the assessment, both Dean and Maxine were the "stars" of their respective families of origin. Dean was the youngest male, doted upon by parents and his sisters, and Maxine was "daddy's girl," and the beauty in her family. But while each partner enjoyed their special status, it was also a problem for them. Maxine felt as if she was special only because of her looks and she felt treated like a sexual object her whole life. She also felt guilty over her father's attention, as if she were like one of the beautiful women he cheated on her mother with.

Dean knew that he was spoiled and could be demanding, but he disliked having to be perfect and to wait to find the perfect mate to please his mother and sisters. He also knew that because he was babied, he did not have the respect of his father. The following is an excerpt depicting how the therapist helped each partner to make the connection between their pasts and their conflict with expectations:

Therapist: It seems as if the two of you have something in common.

Maxine: We both want sex but can't seem to get it?

Therapist: That too, I suppose. But I was thinking about the way you both were treated in your respective families of origin.

Maxine: Oh. Yeah, we were both favored.

Therapist: Right. How do you think that may have affected you both?

Maxine: I think it spoiled us both.

Dean: I guess.

Therapist: Dean, you're not sure?

Dean: I just don't think that I'm asking for too much here.

Maxine: But do you think that you are giving that much?

Dean: I do a lot for you, but you expect me to live without sex.

Maxine: I don't expect either of us to live without it. But I expect you to have some empathy for me. I don't like the situation I'm in any more than you do. But you blame me.

Therapist: It sounds as if you both are saying the same thing: that you both want to be understood. You both are expecting too much from the other given your backgrounds.

Maxine: You mean because we were spoiled?

Therapist: Well, you both were treated as if you were special in your families, but you both had problems with this as well. That's why your expectations are just high enough to fail.

Maxine: Because we are in conflict about getting what we want?

Therapist: Yes. This would make your reactions to each other counterproductive.

Dean: In some ways we both got most of what wanted and in other ways we didn't. We didn't get our fathers' acceptance. So, I can see how we might be confused about what we deserve.

Therapist: Sounds about right.

Step 5. Differentiating from the family of origin to better integrate and balance the couple's conflict.
To help the couple rid themselves of their symptoms and balance their conflict with expectations the case called for a two-front war: Treat the couple's conflict with expectations from a psychodynamic perspective to help each partner

to better differentiate from their respective families of origin, and to eventually integrate sex therapy exercises to alleviate Maxine's vaginismus.

To appropriately differentiate and balance their shared conflict with expectations, Maxine would have had to feel more comfortable with her special status and Dean had to give up some of his. This would no easy task because they have benefited from being stars despite the consequences. Dean was the "golden child" in his family of origin, but he paid the price by acting spoiled, being demanding of others, limiting himself, and by not having the respect of his father. To get his conflict under control and to improve his marriage, he would have to trade some of his status so that he could be more supportive of his wife and to ultimately have his sexual expectations met.

Maxine would have to become more comfortable with her good looks and accept that her mother and others may be jealous of her. But she will also have to own that she has other attributes beyond looks that attract people. In this sense, she would need to come to see that she is lovable beyond her looks and to stop testing Dean. This way she will have her expectations fulfilled without conflict.

As shown below, dilaters of different sizes were prescribed and integrated into the treatment in a graded sequence from smallest to the largest. The successful transfer from the last and largest dilater to Dean's penis was the final formal step in the process of treating Maxine's vaginismus but I recommended two booster sessions following formal termination, six weeks apart for therapeutic maintenance. Keep in mind the couple may increase their sabotaging behavior the closer they get to having their sexual expectations met.

Therapist: It seems that both of you have something to lose if you choose to get your needs met.

Dean: I don't get it.

Therapist: Well, both of you held special or exalted positions in your respective families of origin. Dean, you were the "golden boy" and you Maxine had the looks in the family and were "daddy's girl." And make no mistake about it, this specialness has served both of you well in life. But at what cost?

Dean: I know my dad didn't like it.

Maxine: And I know my mother and siblings were jealous of me. Sometimes I think my looks were a curse.

Therapist: I understand your sentiment, Maxine. Dean, you demand to have your needs met and the more you do the angrier and resistant Maxine gets. Maxine, you have a sexual disorder that you do not have control over, and you have ceased having all sexual intimacy, which is causing Dean to threaten to end the marriage. Dean, do you think your specialness is worth it? Maxine, do you think your discomfort with your looks and insistence that you are only as lovable as your body, is worth it?

Dean: If I knew how to do it, I would give up some of my specialness to get Maxine back.

Maxine: And I hate having vaginismus. I feel so out-of-control.

Therapist: Yes. You are both in a tough situation and compromising with your conflict will be difficult. Our conflicts play hard ball with us. But the upside is tremendous. Dean, you might get more affection and sex from Maxine. And you may even improve your relationship with your father. Maxine, you might be able to rid yourself of your need to see yourself as a one-dimensional person and alleviate your vaginismus.

Maxine: Sounds great to me.

Therapist: Okay. While we are processing this in therapy, we may need to add a few exercises for the vaginismus to help things along. Are you two up for this?

Maxine: Yes.

Therapist: Okay. Now before I assign the first exercise, I want to let you know that because your conflict is about expectations there may be greater resistance just prior to getting them met. This is the way the unconscious conflict is battling to maintain its control over you. But we will deal with that if, and when, it occurs.

Dean: So, what you are saying is that we might sabotage our exercises to maintain the conflict.

Therapist: Yes. Unfortunately, this is all too common. But try it. I think you two are ready. Maxine, I know you can masturbate to orgasm, so are you okay inserting the dilaters yourself or would you prefer Dean to do so? I want you to feel as comfortable as possible.

Maxine: He can do it.

Therapist: Okay. Then lubricate the smallest dilater and Dean gently insert it with a slight twisting motion stopping if Maxine says it is too painful. Maxine you might want to inhale before he inserts the dilater and exhale as he twists it out. Also, rather than focus on what he is doing, think relaxing thoughts if you can. You might even take a warm shower before the exercise if it relaxes you. Try this twice this week and we will meet next week to check your progress.

During the week the couple were able to get through the first exercise with little problem, so we moved to the second dilater using the previous instructions. The session picks up after the second exercise.

Therapist: How did it go?

Dean: Not so good. Maxine got mad at me and would not do the exercise.

Maxine: That's because Dean wanted to skip the second dilater and move to the third one. He wants this all over with. I said no.

Therapist: Dean, you went against my instructions. What was that about?

Dean: I just think this can take forever and I have been waiting for sex forever.

Therapist: So, you think by moving things up will get you sex faster?

Dean: I thought it might work.

Therapist: But it set you back. I suspect that your conflict was unconsciously activated thus preventing you from having your expectations for sex met. Now you are no closer to getting sex from your wife and may be even further away from it.

Maxine: You can say that again. But this is how he treated me before the exercises.

Dean: This is hard.

Therapist: Yes. No pain, no gain. Now try the second dilater again and let's see what happens.

The couple were able to do this exercise twice with little problem. Maxine did report discomfort, but not enough to stop the exercise.

Therapist: So. How did the exercises go?

Maxine: They went well but the second dilater hurt a little.

Therapist: Did you use the lubricant?

Maxine: Yes.

Therapist: Maxine, are you interested in any anti-anxicty medication? It might help you to relax your muscles.

Maxine: No, not yet.

Therapist: Okay. Let's go with the second dilater again but this time lead with the first dilater to stretch the muscle a bit before inserting the second one.

In this third week the couple only partially followed my instructions primarily because of an altercation about what time to do it. This is a common way to sabotage and most often it is better to be as structured with the exercises as possible to avoid too much resistance.

Maxine: Dean scheduled a call with his boss when we had an exercise planned. It made me mad so I would not do the exercise that day.

Dean: I think she blew this one. We had nothing else that day and could have easily rescheduled the exercise. Instead, we could only try it once this past week and Maxine was too tight on the second try for it to work. I think she was still mad at me.

Therapist: Maxine, is that true?

Maxine: Yes. He needs to show me that this is a priority.

Therapist: Could it have really been an important call, and not about you Maxine?

Dean: That's all it was. My boss could only speak at that time. It was nothing personal.

With that explanation we stayed again with the second dilater – preceded by the first. The couple began to see how their sabotaging was only delaying their progress.

Therapist: How did it go this time?

Dean: That idea of using the first dilater as a prep for the second one seemed to work.

Maxine: Yes, it gives me time to get myself ready.

Therapist: Okay. This week try the third dilater but prime yourself with the first and second. And don't forget to use the lubricant.

The couple did well again, and Maxine was especially pleased with her progress. It was still obvious, however, by Dean's body language and somewhat pressured speech that he was in a hurry, but he was controlling himself.

Therapist: How did the exercises go?

Maxine: Great. We're getting there, and Dean has been very gentle with me even though I know it is his nature to be impatient.

Therapist: Dean, how are you doing?

Dean: I'm okay. But I keep having trouble fighting off anger for how long this is taking. I keep having thoughts that I should have left two years agon when this all started.

Therapist: That's interesting Dean. Now that you are on the verge of getting sex you begin to step up your anger and regrets about not leaving Maxine. What do you think this is about?

Dean: I think it's normal. My wife didn't give me sex for two years.

Therapist: Well Dean, we both agree that your feelings are normal. But we do not agree on why they are normal. I think they are normal given your conflict. I think you are trying, with help from your conflict, to prevent yourself from getting sex for the first time in two years.

Dean: Oh, I forgot about the dumb conflict.

Therapist: [Chuckling] It would be easier if it were dumb. So, are you both ready for the last dilater?

Maxine: Let's do it.

The couple were to use the last and largest dilater with lubricant but to first prep with the first three. However, the day before they were to try the exercise, I received a call from Maxine telling me that the couple got into an argument and that Dean had left the house. I told her that this was relatively expected and that I would give him a call. During this call it was apparent that both he and Maxine sabotaged the exercise. Maxine picked on him about looking at another woman when they were out to dinner and Dean told her that another woman wouldn't be so prudish. During the telephone call to Dean, I convinced him to attend the next session with his wife so that we could iron things out. I reiterated that they were so close, and that this is what usually happens especially with this conflict. I was careful to give both partners responsibility for sabotaging the exercise. He reluctantly agreed.

Therapist: So, it sounds as if you two had a rough week.

Maxine: Yup. Dean told me what you said to him, and I guess I blew it as well.

Dean: Man, I see how tough this conflict can be. It messes with both of us.

Therapist: Yes. It sure does. But let's try the exercise again.

This time the exercise went well, and Maxine was relieved. Dean was still skeptical that it could successfully be transferred to his penis, but the couple were able to have intercourse with little discomfort. They then brought up termination.

Therapist: Well, how does it feel to have intercourse again?

Maxine: I am thrilled. I used to think I was sentenced to not having any more sex. I just hope it lasts. And Dean seemed proud of himself.

Dean: Well, I feel like a man again.

Therapist: You were always a man, Dean. Were you able to achieve orgasms?

Maxine: Dean did but not me yet. But I think this will happen since I could before.

Therapist: Okay, great. Keep going. And remember that when you get in trouble, and it is only human that you will, it is your conflict operating. Do not get upset and sabotage yourselves. Conflicts never completely die; they are only manageable. So, flare ups will be a normal occurrence. Hopefully they will be less frequent and less intense and will not result in any lasting symptoms. With regards to termination. I highly recommend that we continue the therapy for a couple more weeks while you continue to have intercourse to make sure the conflict is truly stabilized, and you both are getting your expectations met. If all goes well, we can take a couple of months off and meet again for a booster session or two, if needed.

The couple continued to have intercourse twice weekly and Maxine's comfort grew in direct relation to how Dean treated her and *vice versa*. Both partners were able to control their conflict with little sabotage.

Treating Ken and Sybil: Sexual Symptom – Premature Ejaculation (PE) (See Figure 6.4)

Initial Contact

Ken, a librarian, called to make an appointment for him and his wife of 11 years Sybil, a computer programmer. Ken was 42 years old, and Sybil was 40. The

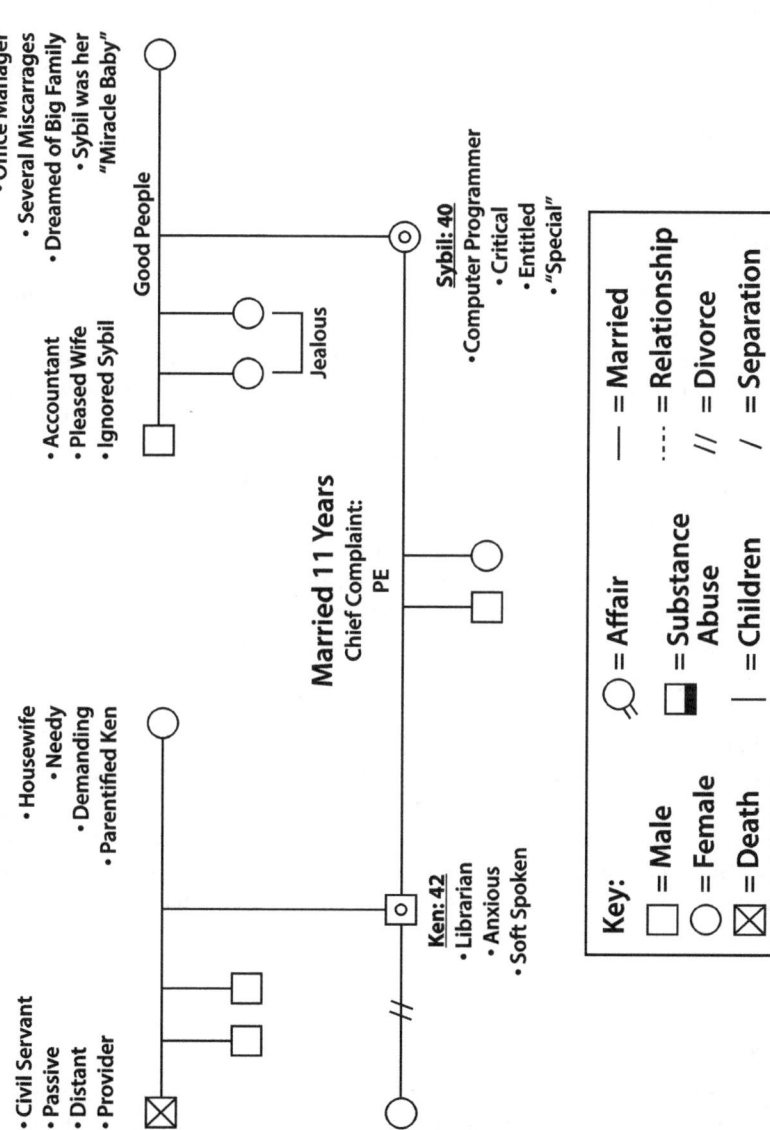

Figure 6.4 Ken and Sybil.

couple had two special needs children. This was Ken's second marriage. Ken claimed that he had never had PE and that Sybil is the first woman to complain. He said that in his first marriage and during his subsequent dating period he would last approximately 10 minutes with continuous thrusting during intercourse. He claimed that his problem developed soon after marriage to Sybil and that now he lasts approximately 2 minutes; sometimes he ejaculates as soon as he penetrates Sybil, before he has a chance to thrust. Ken admitted that Sybil is upset with him in part because she enjoys vaginal orgasms. He admitted that he was very nervous because he feared that Sybil would leave him as his first wife did.

The First Session

Ken presented as a soft spoken, yet anxious man. He claimed that he wanted to please his wife sexually, but his PE prevented this. Sybil was angry and outspoken. She claimed that despite encouraging Ken to seek treatment, he procrastinated and now she feels it's his problem to fix. Ken said that he went to see his urologist when Sybil first complained about his problem; it was the sex therapy that he failed to follow up on. He said that he felt bad about this but that he was afraid to go to a therapist for fear he would be told that it was something that he could not fix.

It was clear in the first session that Sybil was demanding of Ken in more than just a sexual context. She gave the impression that she rescued Ken from the trauma of his first wife leaving him – for another man – and that she felt as if she did him a favor. She could be critical of him as made evident in this session by putting him down whenever he got off point or spoke too slowly. She expected Ken to be thankful to her for marrying him and she said as much. She also expected him to cater to her every need and was not ashamed to admit it.

Ken measured his words. He seemed to vacillate between his open fear of Sybil and by unconsciously retaliating passive aggressively. He would distance as much as possible. True to Sybil's analysis, Ken expected Sybil to make him whole. He said that he liked being married and would never want to be alone again. Ken came off as a powerless man in a desperate situation. There was some concern that if Sybil left him over this problem, he might psychologically deteriorate.

Genogram

Ken was the youngest of three brothers. He described his father as a passive, civil servant who kept to himself. Ken liked his father but did not have much of a relationship with him. He said his father was a solid working man but would spend a great deal of time watching television. According to Ken, his father had no hobbies but was a solid provider. In fact, one of the things he admired his father for was his strong and steady work ethic.

Ken saw his mother as more demanding, especially after his father died of a sudden heart attack. When Ken told the story about his father's death, he showed no emotion. When he was questioned about the tragedy, he said that he "barely knew the man." However, following his father's death, Ken's mother became more needy and demanding and Ken said that he did his best to take care of her. He said that his brothers disappeared, leaving him with all the responsibility, which Ken believes cost him his first marriage. It was then that Ken became fully parentified (Boszormenyi-Nagy & Spark 1973).

Sybil was the youngest of three sisters. She was the baby of the family and treated as if she was special by her mother from the time she was born. Sybil's mother, an office manager at a medical practice, had always wanted a large family and her definition of this was a minimum of three children. After conceiving two daughters there was a series of miscarriages and Sybil was considered the miracle baby that made her mother's dream of a big family come true. Sybil's father was described as an "average guy" who lived to please his wife. He saw Sybil's birth as a relief in that it made his wife happy, but he generally ignored Sybil. He saw her as his wife's daughter. Sybil's father worked as an accountant.

Interactional Style

Sybil was the dominant partner, and the couple could best be described as a confrontational–elusive couple. Ken tried to avoid Sybil's wrath as best he could, but this only made things worse for him. Telling Sybil how scared he was of her only seemed to embolden her; it did not result in a more empathic response from her.

Assessment

Although Ken's father paid little attention to him, his mother had unrealistically high expectations of him as she did for most people around her. Ken was to make her happy. Ken's conflict around expectations was evident in that he was attracted to demanding women and felt it was his job to meet their needs. But he was limited in his capacity to do so and in turn felt burdened by the responsibility. The less he was able to meet their needs, the angrier they became with him. The concept of failing these women frightened him. His father was able to satisfy a demanding woman at least enough for her not to leave him, but Ken took his wife's leaving personally and was now afraid the past would repeat itself.

Ken expected Sybil to help make up for the loss of his first wife. These were unrealistically high expectations. When his first wife left him, he claimed that he was traumatized and felt lost for the longest time. Although he barely had a relationship with his father, he role-modeled him in that he was also a steady worker who always brought home a paycheck. This was, in fact, the way his father was able to keep his marriage together. But Ken's first wife was far more ambitious and wanted more out of Ken than he could provide. When his father died, and he had to take on the responsibility of caring for his demanding mother, she said that she had enough and left him for another man.

Sybil expected that Ken would meet her needs and as mentioned, she expected him to do so in repayment for her rescuing him from the trauma he experienced at the hands of his first wife. But I suspected that Sybil would have been demanding of Ken regardless of his past. And Ken was limited in what he could do for Sybil, and the fear that she might leave him often left him angry and paralyzed with fear.

On the surface it looked as if Sybil had no problem with having her expectations fulfilled. And it was evident that her mother had unrealistically high expectations for her as the "miracle baby." But this exalted position came with a price. She was hated by both of her jealous sisters and ignored by her father. Her demanding nature also cost her relationships with friends and suitors. Sybil's conflict around expectations was made evident in that although she demanded that her needs be met, she chose a man, Ken, who had limited resources and was ambivalent about being a caretaker. And she could be critical, rather than providing Ken with much needed support and positive reinforcement so that he could better meet her needs. The way Sybil treated Ken made it less likely that he could meet her expectations.

Ken had acquired PE with no other significant sexual issues. There was no history of abuse on either partner's part and no fetishes or paraphilias. Ken did find that Sybil was more aggressive than other women he has been with during foreplay. He claimed that he asked her to be more patient with him, but this angered her. Ken did masturbate 1–2 times per week, but he claimed that he only fantasized about having sex with Sybil. He said that he still came relatively quickly (i.e., approximately 4–5 minutes), but not as fast as he does with Sybil.

Sybil was not on any medication. Ken was prescribed the SSRI paroxetine hydrochloride (Paxil), but this did not help to delay his ejaculation. He had not tried condoms for fear he might lose his erection, which he self-rated a healthy 8 or 9 in terms of firmness (Kaplan, personal communication, October 7, 1987). Ken had seen a therapist for a short time after his first wife had left him. A psychiatrist associated with his therapist first prescribed Paxil, but Ken eventually stopped seeing him and allowed his family doctor to continue prescribing this medication.

Treatment

Step 1. Determining the couple's expectations and their connection to the couple's symptoms.

It seemed clear that Ken was dependent on Sybil to bolster his self-esteem and self-worth, especially given the trauma of his first wife leaving him. He expected Sybil to make up for his loss, stabilize him, and give him a sense of security. In return, he did what his father did: he went to work every day and paid the bills. But Sybil wanted much more. She wanted more money, more excitement, and great sex.

The biggest challenge in this case was convincing the couple that their unmet expectations were connected in any way to Ken's PE. While Ken claimed to be willing to do the work to please Sybil, Sybil had difficulty taking any responsibility for her contribution to Ken's PE. She was adamant that it was Ken's problem. The following excerpt shows how the couple were helped to make the connection between their shared conflict with expectations and the PE symptom:

Therapist: Ken, I believe that Sybil is right that you are dependent on her to help you to heal from your first marriage.

Ken: She is, but I also do love her. I don't want another divorce.

Sybil: That's what you are going to get if you don't do something about your problem.

Therapist: How do you feel when you hear that, Ken?

Ken: Really scared. I'm doing all I can.

Therapist: But does hearing that help you in any way?

Ken: I don't know. Sybil does need to kick me in the butt from time to time, but it does frighten me. I just keep thinking she's going to leave me and it's harder to concentrate.

Therapist: So overall its more of a problem than a solution?

Ken: Yes. I'm too afraid that I will let her down. I think that's why I procrastinated.

Sybil: I don't want to hear any more excuses.

Therapist: I get it Sybil. And I am not debating your feelings. I just find it interesting that the way you are trying to help might be working against you.

Sybil: What do you mean?

Therapist: Well, I think that Ken needs positive reinforcement and support with this problem. Criticism is obviously scaring him, and it will probably make it harder for him to get control of it.

Sybil: How would you feel?

Therapist: Again, I am not challenging your feelings. Your tactics are working against you. And if you want to rid yourself of this problem there might be a more productive way.

Step 2. Exposing the couple's conflict with having their expectations met.
While it was hard for both partners to accept that they were working against themselves, especially Sybil, whose anger and defensiveness proved to be destructive. Ken's contribution came in the form of his fear and powerlessness. The following brief exchange shows how the therapist helped the couple see their shared conflict:

Sybil: I am upset with you because you seem to think that I don't want Ken to get over his PE.

Therapist: I can see that. But I just want you to meet your needs.

Sybil: So, you really think I not trying to get my needs met. Why?

Therapist: I suspect you are acting at cross purposes because you may be in conflict about having your expectations met. Why else would you be doing something that prevents you from getting what you say you want?

Sybil: But I am trying to push Ken to meet my needs.

Therapist: And if it worked, I would be all for it. But it is working in reverse. Even Ken admitted as much. And you have incredibly high standards; some might consider them unrealistic. These are the signs of a conflict: when someone is working hard for something and continuously achieving the opposite of what they claim to expect. But I am not giving you full responsibility here Sybil. Ken, you say that you will do anything to please Sybil and fear going through another divorce. Yet you procrastinated in seeking sex therapy and at every turn you give your personal power away by being so scared and reliant on Sybil. You also chose to marry a woman with very high standards, and I am not so sure you were prepared to meet them even before the onset of PE. I suspect you too are in conflict about having your expectations met.

Ken: I see that. I guess I haven't made it easy on myself either.

Step 3. Broadening the context of the couple's conflict with expectations.
Sybil was demanding outside of the context of the couple's PE. As mentioned, she wanted more money and a more exciting life. Ken, however, wasn't nearly as ambitious. He was steady and stable, and every day was the same for him. He was confused as to why Sybil would bring such drama to their plain but serene lives. The following exchange demonstrates how the couple's context was broadened to show Sybil how demanding she could be in general and how Ken's sense of powerlessness existed in other contexts:

Therapist: Ken, do you think that Sybil has high standards?

Ken: Well, I don't want to make her angry.

Sybil: (Sarcastically) Go on Ken, say something. The therapist will protect you.

Ken: Yes, Sybil is tough.

Therapist: How do you feel about what Sybil just said?

Ken: I don't know.

Therapist: Sybil said you can speak your mind.

Ken: I think it was mean. But she does have a right to be angry with me.

Therapist: Because of the PE?

Ken: Yes.

Therapist: Do you think she is angry about anything else?

Ken: Well, the money.

Sybil: I think what he means is he has been passed over for many promotions. He is just so passive.

Therapist: Sybil, what Ken does for a living historically does not pay very well. Do you really think you would be satisfied if he were given a raise?

Sybil: Probably not. But it would be better than it is now.

Therapist: But not enough to quell your anger and disappointment. And Ken, why don't you apply for promotions?

Ken: I don't like to push my employers. I could end up losing my job.

Therapists: So, you're afraid of them too?

Ken: I guess.

Step 4. Determining the origin of the couple's conflict with expectations.

It was hard for Ken to connect his internal conflict to his attraction to demanding women and his inability to meet their needs. He was not a man of insight. Sybil was too defended in her anger to accept the connection, but she gave the impression that she was a smart woman who still believed it was easier to rely on others to meet her needs than to take them on herself. She also did not seem to be interested in exploring her impact on her sisters and the absent relationship with her father. The following excerpt shows how the therapist helped the couple to connect their shared conflict with expectations to their respective families of origin:

Therapist: Ken would you say that you are an ambitious man?

Ken: (Chuckling) No, not at all.

Therapist: Yet you tend to surround yourself with women who have pretty high standards.

Ken: I sure do, don't I?

Therapist: Yes. And it doesn't sound as if your father role modeled ambition either.

Ken: No. He was a regular guy. But he was steady. He held the same job for years and rarely missed a day's work. He was a solid provider.

Therapist: Was your mother satisfied with the lifestyle he provided her with?

Ken: I think so. I mean she never said anything about it.

Therapist: What is so attractive to you about demanding women?

Ken: Beats me.

Sybil: We get things done. We are the movers and shakers. Half the stuff we have and do are my ideas. He would just sit in front of the television all night if it were up to him.

Ken: Yeah. I guess I don't need much.

Therapist: On the contrary. I agree with Sybil. You desperately need a strong woman. You expect her to push you, and yet you also expect her to accept your limitations. But this is an unrealistically high expectation because the strong women you choose – including Sybil – do not seem to like limitations. You can work hard to try and please them. But can they be pleased?

Ken: So, you think I am working hard to please Sybil, but she may never allow herself to be pleased?

Therapist: Yes. Because you and Sybil share the same conflict about getting your collective needs met. Sybil was the "miracle baby" of her household, but she is in conflict about that, aren't you Sybil?

Sybil: I am not sure I know what you mean.

Therapist: You do not see the connection between growing up special and how demanding you are?

Sybil: Okay. I can buy that. I heard it from my siblings growing up.

Therapist: Great. All I am adding here is that you also felt other feelings as well.

Sybil: Yes. I was angry. I felt picked on.

Therapist: Right. And you had no relationship with your father.

Sybil: Yes. That still hurts.

Therapist: Now we are getting somewhere.

Step 5. Differentiating from the family of origin to better integrate and balance the couple's conflict.

To help the couple rid themselves of their symptoms and balance their conflict with expectations this case also called for a two-front war: Treat the couple's conflict with expectations while integrating sex therapy exercises to alleviate Ken's PE.

To appropriately differentiate and balance their shared conflict with expectations, Sybil, like Maxine, would have had to feel more comfortable with her special status, but Ken would have to deal with his attitude about pleasing women versus the burden he feels when he enters what he perceives as an impossible mission.

Specifically, Sybil would have to give up, in her mind, some of the status she was accorded in her family of origin and keep in mind what it cost her: alienation from her father and siblings; and the passivity of her husband, Ken. She might then be able to be kinder and less demanding of Ken, which will make it easier for him to meet her expectations. Ken would have to regulate his feelings of being burdened by women, which will enable him to be less ambivalent and fatalistic about meeting their needs. This will in turn reduce the pressure on him and he will be more likely to get his needs met. Let us now see how sex therapy exercises were integrated into the psychodynamic treatment of Ken and Sybil.

The stop-start technique (Semans, 1956; Kaplan, 1974; Betchen & Gambesica, 2020) was found useful in treating Ken's PE, especially because of his anxiety and Sybil's anger. After softening up the couple's defenses, I believed that exercises might have a positive impact. First, Ken was prescribed individual masturbatory exercises which progressed to partner masturbatory exercises, and eventually to a modified form of intercourse. The following exchange depicts how these exercises were integrated into Ken and Sybil's therapy and linked to the couple's shared conflict with expectations that emanated from each partner's family of origin. The example also illustrates how the couples therapist dealt with each partner's resistances:

Therapist: Do either of you have any objections to trying a few exercises for your PE? It seems to me that although you still might be somewhat skeptical, you seem to be accepting of the possibility that a conflict with expectations is operating.

Ken: I'm ready.

Sybil: We have nothing to lose at this point. Things can't get that much worse.

Therapist: Let's find out. Ken, begin by trying to relax, perhaps take a warm shower, and turn off your cell phone. Lie on your bed without clothes or at least without your pants and begin to stroke yourself. Pay attention to your feelings, especially when you are feeling aroused. When you get to the point that you feel you are about to ejaculate, stop stroking and let that immediate sensation go away. Do not, however, let your erection disappear. As soon as the feeling subsides repeat the exercise four times. If you feel like having an orgasm on the fourth time, feel free to do so. Try this exercise 3–4 times this week and in the next session we will talk about it. Sybil, if you wish Ken to pleasure you, he can before the exercise.

Sybil: That's okay. I'll wait.

In the following session, Ken reported that he did the exercise twice during the week, not the prescribed four times. He said the couple were too busy. But he reported that all went well and that he was able to control his ejaculation for about five minutes the first time, and seven minutes the second time. He admitted that even though he thought about Sybil while he was pleasuring himself, he did not feel the pressure that he does when he is with her. Just as a precaution, I asked Ken to repeat the exercise three more times before the next session. The dialogue will pick up after this assignment:

Therapist: How did the exercises go, Ken?

Ken: They went well. I lasted eight minutes with continuous masturbating the last time.

Therapist: Great. Are you ready for partner exercises?

Ken: If Sybil is?

Sybil: Okay, what do we do?

Therapist: Try the same exercise but this time Sybil, you do the stroking. Ken, when you are getting close to the point of ejaculation, give Sybil a signal to let up. Ken, if at that point you can get by with Sybil holding onto your penis, fine. But if you can't let Sybil know so she can remove her hand from your penis. Sybil, only resume stroking when Ken tells you that it's okay. Got that?

Ken: Yes.

The couple, as is often the case, ran into some problems with the partner exercises.

Sybil: Well, we could only do the exercise once and that didn't go so well. Ken didn't give me enough time to stop stroking him, so he could not hold off for more than a few seconds. Then he didn't want to try it again.

Therapist: What happened Ken?

Ken: I don't know.

Therapist: That's interesting. You did fine on your own, but we included Sybil, you had difficulty. What do you think the difference is?

Ken: I don't know. I am more nervous when Sybil is around because I'm afraid that I will fail and make her angry.

Sybil: So, you think giving up will make me happy?

Therapist: Tell me more about that, Ken

Ken: I can't explain it, but I go into a fog.

Therapist: The pressure is on.

Ken: Yes.

Therapist: That's natural, but I don't think this is all about pressure. What else are you feeling?

Ken: There is a part of me that doesn't want to do this, but I really do want to make Sybil happy.

Therapist: It's a lot of work, isn't it? I mean to make someone happy.

Ken: Yes.

Therapist: It's especially hard if you're not even sure it will work. Have you ever felt that way before?

Ken: Yes. With my mother. I wanted to run away. I was caught between my obligation to make her happy and wanting to escape. And mom would get angry with me if I didn't meet her expectations.

Therapist: But as Sybil pointed out, giving up doesn't seem to work either. Did you ever give up on your mother?

Ken: I couldn't. I'd feel too guilty.

Therapist: Sounds like a double bind. If you work on pleasing someone and you can't, it is frustrating and potentially detrimental to the relationship, but there may be severe consequences if you give up. That's a tough place to be.

Ken: Yeah, and Sybil has been in a bad mood.

Sybil: I hadn't been feeling well. I doubt that's the conflict on my part.

Therapist: Maybe. We'll see. Try the exercise again twice this coming week.

This time Sybil got mad at Ken about something unrelated to their sexual problem and refused to do the exercise. Ken was decidedly nervous about this. He saw every one of Sybil's resistances as a sign she was about to leave him. What he was really doing, however, was unconsciously making himself nervous so that he could not meet his or Sybil's expectations.

Therapist: What happened this week, Sybil?

Sybil: Ken upset me. He was supposed to clean the garage this past weekend. He has been promising me he would do it for months. And I finally snapped. I wasn't about to do those exercises with him.

Therapist: That's interesting Sybil. You say that you are the one who wants this PE treated. And yet you found a way to sabotage the exercise. Are you sure that you want to have vaginal orgasms again?

Sybil: I do. But it's hard to separate the sexual from the nonsexual.

Therapist: It's especially difficult if you have a conflict with getting your expectations met. Remember, only a part of you wants to be a star and to get your needs met. The other part of you is uncomfortable with it. Let's try this exercise again.

The couple were able to get through the partner stroking stop-start exercise, but Ken was having trouble. He was ejaculating after a couple of strokes. The following will demonstrate why:

Therapist: What happened with the exercise?

Sybil: Ken has no control.

Therapist: What do you think would help you, Ken?

Ken: It would help if Sybil would slow her stoking down. She grabs me and strokes so hard and fast I can't control myself. I think she's trying to make me lose control.

Therapist: What's that about Sybil?

Sybil: Okay. I know. I sabotaged this time. It's so weird. These exercises are here to help me too, but I screwed them up.

Therapist: It's not easy to give up even a small bit of your star power even though it has cost you.

The couple were finally successful. We repeated the stroking one more week and moved to another exercise.

Therapist: Ken, now that you are lasting through five minutes of Sybil stroking you, I think we can move on. Sybil, are you still sure that you do not want Ken to please you before the exercise?

Sybil: I'm good.

Therapist: Okay. But is it possible that your conflict is enabling you to reject being pleasured?

Sybil: I'll have to think about that one.

Therapist: Okay. Sybil for this exercise straddle Ken and apply the same the start-stop exercise.

The couple had to repeat this exercise for three consecutive weeks. In the first week Ken sabotaged his focus. In the second week, Sybil went back to stroking too hard and too quickly. Every sabotage was framed as an unconscious way to prevent the couple from having their sexual expectations met and connected back to their respective families of origin. By the third week the couple settled down and successfully completed the exercise.

Therapist: I think we are ready for the next exercise. Assume the same position with Sybil on top. But this time Sybil, instead of stroking Ken, rub his penis against the opening of your vagina. Ken, give yourself enough time to stop Sybil when you sense that you are about to lose control.

Ken: Okay.

The couple did well with this exercise and Ken was able to last 6–7 minutes of continuous rubbing. Sybil was optimistic, but she tried to kill her optimism with "what ifs."

Ken: That went well. But Sybil is starting to worry about what will happen if this doesn't work. She's upsetting me.

Therapist: I suspect you are at it again Sybil.

Sybil: Maybe. But I can't help it.

Therapist: Yes. Your conflict is a tough hombre. It will not give into you without a fight. You will have to consider it when you are getting anxious. That is, immediately think of whether you are trying to reduce your chances of getting your expectations met.

Sybil gained some control over her pessimism and the exercise proved successful when reassigned. Next the couple were to try intercourse using the "quiet vagina" technique (Hartman & Fithian, 1972).

Therapist: Okay. Sybil, the next exercise entails you sitting on top of Ken again and rubbing his penis against your vagina. Once he is hard enough for penetration mount him and insert his penis inside you slowly and gently. After insertion do not move at first. Give Ken some time to acclimate. When he gives you the word that he feels in control, move slowly until he again reaches the point right before he is about to ejaculate and then immediately stop and remain still. Resume movement when he gives the okay. Got it?

Sybil: Got it. But suppose he loses it as soon as he enters me?

Therapist: Don't worry about it. Just go slow.

Sybil sabotaged this exercise. According to Ken she hopped on top of him and began thrusting fast and hard. He lasted 15 seconds. When confronted Sybil was defensive.

Therapist: What happened with the exercise?

Ken: Sybil went crazy on me. I don't think anyone could have withstood that attack.

Sybil: I don't know what came over me. I lost it.

Therapist: I think the conflict came over you. You're close to getting what you have been asking for. And remember, because your mother gave you everything that you desired, your siblings hated you and your father distanced from you.

Sybil: That was such a weird thing. I did get a little anxious. I guess I sabotaged the exercise.

Therapist: Try it again.

The exercise went well and was reassigned for good measure. Ken was consistently lasting for approximately six minutes, and so the couple were told to do repeat the exercise until they were able to last 8–10 minutes. They reached this goal with only a few glitches, completed the exercise, and terminated treatment. However, as is usually the case, I predicted that the conflict would strike at random times and the couple needed to be prepared for this. I called them two months following formal termination to see if they required a booster session to find out that they were still doing well, but because they had some difficulty, Ken decided to wear a condom to cut down even further on his sensitivity. Sybil did not mind. She said that she would have considered it sabotaging to object.

References

Addar, M. H. (2004). The unconsummated marriage: causes and Management. *Clinical and Experimental Obstetrics & Gynecology, 31*, 279–281.

Alizadeh, A., Farnam, F., Raisi, F., & Parsaeian, M. (2019). Prevalence of risk factors for genito-pelvic pain/penetration disorder: A population-based study of Iranian women. *Journal of Sexual Medicine, 16*, 1068–1077.

American Psychiatric Association (2013). *Diagnostic and statistical manual of mental disorders* (5th ed.). Author.

Amidu, N., Owiredu, W. K., Woode, E., Addai-Mensah, O., Quaye, L., Alhassan, A., & Tagoe, E. A. (2010). Incidence of sexual dysfunction: a prospective survey in Ghanaian females. *Reproductive Biology and Endocrinology, 8*, 1–6. doi: 10.1186/1477-7827-8-106. PMID: 20809943.

Asimakopolous, A., Miano, R., Agro, E. F., Vespasiani, G., & Spera, E. (2012). Does current. scientific and clinical evidence support the use of phosphodiesterase type 5 inhibitors for the treatment of premature ejaculation? A systematic review and meta-analysis. *Journal of Sexual Medicine, 9*, 2404–2416. doi: 10.1111/jsm.2012.9.issue-9/issuetoc

Avery-Clark, C., & Weiner, L. (2018, July). *Sensate focus: The alchemy of touch, mindfulness & somatic therapy*. Training sponsored by The Integrative Sex Therapy Institute, Training Program, Washington, DC.

Ballard, J. (2021). Relationships: How long should you wait before having sex, moving in together, and getting engaged. YouGovAmerica. Retrieved from https://today.yougov.com/topics/society/articles-reports/2021/08/03/relationships-dating-marriage-sex-milestones-poll

Barbonetti. S., D'Andrea, F., Cavallo, F., Martorella, S., Francavilla, S., & Francavilla, F. (2019). Erectile dysfunction and premature ejaculation in homosexual and heterosexual men: A systemic review and meta-analysis of comparative studies. *The Journal of Sexual Medicine, 16*, 624–632. doi: 10.1016/j.jsxm.2019.02.014

Berenger-Soler, M., Navarro-Sanchez, A., Compañ-Rosique, A., Luri-Preto, P., Navarro-Ortiz, R., Gómez-Pérez, L., Pérez-Tomás, C., Font-Juliá, E., Gil-Gullén, V. F., Cortés-Castell, E., Navarro-Cremades, F., Montejo, A. L., Arroyo-Sebastián, M. D. A., & Pérez-Jover, V. (2022). Genito-pelvic pain/penetration disorder (GPPPD) in Spanish women-clinical approach in primary health care: Review and Meta-analysis. *Journal of Clinical Medicine, 11*, 1–14. doi: 10.3390/jcm1192340

Betchen, S. (2010, July 27). Vaginismus: A most challenging problem. *Psychology Today*. www.psychologytoday.com/us/node/45793/preview

Betchen, S. (2022). *Couples in conflict: Clinical techniques for navigating sexual and relational control struggles*. Routledge.

Betchen, S., & Davidson, H. (2018). *Master conflict therapy: A new model for practicing couples and sex therapy*. Routledge.

Betchen, S., & Gambescia, N. (2020). A new systemic treatment model for couples with premature ejaculation: Master Conflict Theory. In K. Hertlein, N. Gambescia, & G. Weeks (Eds.), *Systemic sex therapy* (3rd ed., pp. 77–91). Routledge.

Bond, K. S., Mpofu, E., & Millington, M. (2015). Treating women with genito-pelvic pain/penetration disorder: Influences of patient agendas on help-seeking. *Journal of Family Medicine, 2*, 1–8.

Borg, C., de Jong, P. J., & Weijmar Schultz, W. (2011). Vaginismus and dyspareunia: Relationship with general and sex-related moral standards. *Journal of Sexual Medicine, 8*, 223–31. doi: 10.1111/j.1743-6109.2010.02080. x

Boszormenyi, N., & Spark, G. (1973). *Invisible loyalties*. Harper & Row.

Brody, S. (2010), The relative health benefits of different sexual activities. *Sexual Medicine, 7*, 1336–1361. https://doi.org/10.1111/j.1743-6109.2009.01677x

Burri, A., Giuliano, F., McMahon, C., & Porst, H. (2014). Female partner's perception of premature ejaculation and its impact on relationship breakups, relationship quality, and sexual satisfaction. *Sexual Medicine, 11*, 2243–55. doi: 10.1111/jsm.12551

Cheng, Z., & Smyth, R. L. (2015). Sex and happiness. *Journal of Economic Behavior & Organization, 112*, 26–32. https://doi.org/10.1016/j.jebo.2014/1.2.630

Fertel, E., Meana, M., & Maykut, C. (2020). Painful intercourse: Genito-pelvic pain penetration disorder. In In K. Hertlein, N. Gambescia, & G. Weeks (Eds.), *Systemic sex therapy* (3rd ed., pp. 145–159). Routledge.

Fiala, L., Lenz, J., Konecna, P., Zajicova, M., Cerna, J., & Sajdlova, R. (2021). *Andrologia, 53*, 14093. doi: 10.1111/and.14093

Freud, S. (1905/1953). Three essays on the theory of sexuality. In J. Strachey (Ed. & Trans.),*The standard edition of the complete psychological works of Sigmund Freud* (Vol. 7, pp. 127–245). London: Hogarth Press and the Institute of Psychoanalysis.

Gök-e, A. F., Demirtas, A., & Ekmekcioglu, O. (2010). The effects of three phosphodiesterace type 5 inhibitors on ejaculation latency time in lifelong premature ejaculators: A double-bind laboratory setting study. *BJU International, 107*, 1274–1277. doi: 10.1111/j.1464-410X.2010.09646.x

Hartman, W. E., & Fithian, M. A. (1972). *Treatment of sexual dysfunction: A bio-psycho-social Approach.* Center for Marital and Sexual Studies.

Hellstrom, W. J. G. (2010). Update of treatment of premature ejaculation. *International Journal of Clinical Practice, 65*, 16–26. doi: 10.1111/jcp2010.65.issue-1/issuetoc

Herbenick, D., Fu, T., Arter, J., Sanders, S., & Dodge, B. (2018). Women's experiences with genital touching, sexual pleasure, and orgasm: results from a U.S. probability sample of women ages 18-94. *Journal of Sex & Marital Therapy, 44*, 201–212. doi: 10.1080/092623X.2017.1346530

International Society for Sexual Medicine (2015). *ISSM quick reference guide to PE*. https://issm.info/media/attachments/2021/08/17/03-clinical-guidelines---issm-quick-reference-guide-to-pe—vjan2015.pdf

Kaplan, H. S. (1974). *The new sex therapy: Active treatment of sexual dysfunctions.* Times Books.

Kerner, I. (2009). *She comes first: The thinking man's guide to pleasuring a woman.* Collins.

Kinsey, A., Pomeroy, W., Martin, C., & Gebhard, P. (1953). *Sexual behavior in the human female.* W. B. Saunders Company.

Kontula, O., & Miettinen, A. (2016). Determinants of female sexual orgasms. *Socioaffective Neuroscience & Psychology, 6*, 1–21. doi: 10.3402/snp.v6.31624

Marchand, E. (2021). Psychological and behavioral treatment of female orgasmic disorder. *Sexual Medicine Reviews, 9*, 194–211. https://doi.org/10.1016/j.sxmr.2020.07.007

Masters, W., & Johnson, V. (1966). *Human sexual response.* Little, Brown, & Company.

Masters, W., & Johnson, V. (1970). *Human sexual inadequacy.* Little, Brown, & Company.

Maximets, N. (2022). Sexless marriage & divorce? When to walk away. OnlineDivorce. Retrieved from https://onlinedivorce.com/blog/sexless-marriage-or-divorce-when-to- walk-away/

McNabney, S. M., Weseman, C., Hevesi, K., & Rowland, D. (2022). Are the criteria for the diagnosis of premature ejaculation applicable to gay men or sexual activities other than penile-vaginal intercourse? *Journal of Sexual Medicine, 10*, 1–13. doi: 10.1016/j.esxm.2022.100516

Mercer, C.H., Prah, P., Field, N., Tanton, C., Macdowall, W., Clifton, S., Hughes, G., Nardone, A., Wellings, K., Johnson, A., & Sonnenberg, P. (2016). The health and well-being of men who have sex with men (MSM) in Britain: Evidence from the third National Survey of Sexual Attitudes and Lifestyles (Natsal-3). *BMC Public Health, 16*, 525. https://doi.org/10.1186/s12889-016-3149-z

Mintz, L. (2018). *Becoming cliterate: Why orgasm equality matters-and how to get it.* HarperOne.

Monsesi, J., Fauber, R., Gordon, E., & Hemberg, R. (2010). The specific importance of communicating about sex to couples' sexual and overall relationship satisfaction. *Journal of Social and Personal Relationships*, *28*, 591–609. https://doi.org/10.1177/026554075 1036833

Nagoski, E. (2021). *Come as you are: The surprising new science that will transform your sex life*. Simon & Schuster.

Raveendran, A. V., & Agarwal, A. (2021). Premature ejaculation—current concepts in the management: A narrative review. *International Journal of Biomedical Research*, *19*, 5–22. doi: 10.18502/ijrm.v19.8176

Roazen, P. (2018). (Ed.). *Helene Deutsch: Psychoanalysis of the sexual functions of women*. Routledge.

Ross, J. (1995). Social class tensions within families. *The American Journal of Family Therapy*, 23, 338–350. https://doi.org/10.1080/01926189508251364

Rowland, D. L., & Kolba, T. N. (2018). The burden of sexual problems: Perceived effects on men's and women's sexual partners. *The Journal of Sex Research*, *55*, 226–235. doi: 10.1080/00224499.2017. 1332153

Rowland, D. L., Kostelyka, K. A., & Tempela, A. R. (2016). Attribution patterns in men with sexual problems: Analysis and implications for treatment. *Sexual & relationship Therapy*, *31*, 148–158. Doi: 10.1080/14681994.2015.1126669

Semens, J. (1956). Premature ejaculation: A new approach. *Southern Medical Journal*, *49*, 353–358. doi: 10.1097/00007611-195604000-00008

Stuparu, C. (2020). Female orgasm, anorgasmia. *International Journal for Advanced Studies in Sexology*, *2*, 89–93. doi: 10.46388/ijass.2020.13.25

Superdrug Online Doctor (2022). It's not you, it's not me—it's ED. Retrieved from https://onlinedoctor.superdrug.com/women-and-ed/

Twenge, J., Sherman, R., & Wells, B. (2017). Declines in sexual frequency among American adults, 1989–2014. *Archives of Sexual Behavior*, *46*, 2389–2401. doi.10.1007/s/0508-017-9553-1

van Lankveld, J. J. D. M., Granot, M., Weijmar Schultz, W. C., Binik, Y., M., Wessleman, U., Pukall, C. F., & Achtrari, C. (2010). Women's sexual pain disorders, *Journal of Sexual Medicine*, *7*, 615–631. https://doi.org/10.1111/j.1743.6109.2009.01631.x

Verze, P., Arcaniolo, D., Imbimbo, C., Cai, T., Venturino, L., Spirito, L.,…Mirone, V. (2018). General and sex profile of women and partner affected by premature ejaculation: Results of a large observational, non-interventional, cross-sectional and epidemiological study (IPER-F). *Andrology*, 6, 714–719. doi: 10.1111/andr.12545

Waldinger, M. (2013). Treatment of premature ejaculation with selective serotonin re-uptake inhibitors. In E. Jannini, C. McMahon, & M. Waldinger (Eds.), *Premature ejaculation: From etiology to diagnosis and treatment* (pp. 229–240). Springer-Verlag.

Weiner, L., & Avery-Clark, C. (2014). *Sensate focus in sex therapy*. Routledge.

Yasan, A., Tamam, L., Ozkan, M., & Gurgen, F. (2009). Premarital sexual attitudes and experiences in university students. *Anatolian Journal of Clinical Investigation*, *3*(3), 174–184.

7   The Therapist's Expectations

More than any other model of psychotherapy, psychoanalysis has emphasized the need for the therapist to undergo personal treatment. In *Analysis Terminable and Interminable*, Freud (1937/1964) wrote:

> Every analyst should periodically – at intervals – of five years or so submit himself to an analysis once more, without feeling ashamed of taking this step. This would mean, then, that not only the therapeutic analysis of patients but his own analysis would change from a terminable into an interminable task.
>
> (p. 249)

Freud was not implying that an analysis should go on forever. He was suggesting that the ending of an analysis was not always clear in part, because an analysis does not aim for human perfection. He wrote: "The business of the analysis is to secure the best possible psychological conditions for the functions of the ego; with that it has discharged its task" (p. 250).

Psychoanalyst Frieda Fromm-Reichmann (1950) added: "any attempt at intensive psychotherapy is fraught with danger, hence unacceptable, where not preceded by the future psychiatrist's personal analysis" (p. 240).

Given MCT's psychoanalytic bent and the importance it places on the motivations of the unconscious mind, it would be helpful for the couples therapist using this model to have experienced a course of personal psychotherapy. This is important so the therapist does not unconsciously interfere with the treatment process or further unbalance the couple's conflict with expectations. If the therapist's own conflict is unbalanced or out-of-control, the therapist may collude with the couple in vacillating – in intensity and frequency – between promoting the couple's expectations while simultaneously sabotaging them. If the therapist has not experienced a course of personal psychotherapy, he or she should endeavor to be aware of any personal conflicts to prevent damaging countertransference issues. The following are some ways in which the therapist's unbalanced conflict with expectations can be to the detriment of both therapist and couple.

DOI: 10.4324/9781003359470-10

The Therapist's Failure to Structure Treatment

All therapists want couples to keep their scheduled appointments, behave in a civil manner in sessions, and to pay their fees. Structuring treatment has proven to be an essential ingredient in achieving a positive therapeutic outcome (Weeks et al., 2005). Without an understanding of his or her personal conflict, the therapist is less likely to structure the treatment process and to meet these expectations. This might be especially true in couples therapy, considered the hardest treatment to practice effectively (Doherty, 2002). Without structure, the couples therapist may easily activate the couple's conflict and enable them to fail to show up for appointments or forget to pay their fees. Partners may even get physical with one another in the heat of the moment. Here are some examples of a lack of therapeutic structure enabled by a couples therapist to the detriment of both therapist and couple:

A trainee at a clinic confessed that although she wanted to collect her fees immediately following her sessions, she felt guilty doing so, often letting weeks go by without payment. While most of her clients paid when asked, there were several times when certain clients resented the large bills they were presented with and refused to pay; others claimed to have paid when they didn't.

Despite her own paralysis, the trainee said that she could not believe that certain couples had the audacity and the lack of integrity to cheat her out of her hard-earned fees. She said that she expected her clients to recognize that she was doing them a favor by being flexible about collecting her fees, and to honor their commitment to the treatment process. Instead, she said, they were acting self-ishly. It was clear the therapist was struggling with a conflict with expectations. She expected her fees to be paid but because she had trouble being assertive, she hoped that the clients would take the initiative or at least pay when presented with the bill.

The Therapist's Expectation of Reciprocity

A therapist may compromise to accommodate a couple. But the therapist who expects this to indebt the couple and gain their undivided loyalty, should con-sider that his/her personal conflict is out of balance. In fact, a situation such as this could backfire, with the client getting used to special considerations from the therapist and expecting it henceforth. For example, a therapist took exten-sive emails and telephone calls from the wife of a couple who she saw as an aggressive, controlling partner who was hard to please. The therapist thought that by allowing this woman to breach therapeutic boundaries she could curry her favor. But this strategy backfired because with every breach, the woman became even more demanding, and eventually the therapist felt completely out of control in the treatment process. Even worse, when the husband found out the extent to which his wife and the therapist were in contact outside of the sessions, he terminated the treatment. The wife then blamed the therapist for ruining her marriage.

Another trainee expected her clients to act civil to one another; to at least keep their hands to themselves during sessions. She said that she trusted her clients to respect the therapeutic process. This turned out to be pollyannaish given how volatile couples therapy can be. In one session, the husband of a couple leaned over and kicked his wife's leg when she said something he didn't like. The therapist did not approve of his retaliation but because no one had ever been physical in her sessions she expressed only mild displeasure and moved on with the treatment. Unfortunately, this conscious oversight enabled the husband to think that his inappropriate behavior would be tolerated, and he took the liberty to throw a Kleenex box at his wife, striking her in the head. In shock, the therapist said that she never expected something like that to happen, especially since she had overlooked the last incident. Her personal conflict with expectations allowed her to expect too much of this man.

The Therapist's Misplaced Empathy

Therapists are famous for their empathy. And while this is a great asset to have as a clinician, it can also lead to therapeutic unbalance, especially in couples therapy. For example, in working with couples, one partner often presents as the perpetrator and the other the victim. While systemic theory posits that each partner makes some contribution to the relationship difficulty, often the partner that is overtly angry, accusatory, or outspoken is given the role of the perpetrator while the meeker, passive partner is seen as the bullied victim. If the couples therapist takes sides and feels compelled to aggressively defend the weaker partner, systemic perspective is lost, and the treatment process is in jeopardy (Weeks & Fife, 2014). Overtly challenging the perceived stronger partner in couples therapy is also dangerous and often ends in premature termination (Betchen, 2005).

While forming a coalition or taking the side of one partner in couples therapy is a problem in itself, it is especially problematic when the therapist expects that because he/she has defended the weaker client, the weaker client will defend the therapist against the more assertive partner. This is an unrealistic expectation and further evidence of a therapist in conflict. The weaker partner usually will not reciprocate, and the therapist's expectations will go unmet (Betchen, 2005). Growing up in a tough neighborhood, it was common for my friends to complain about their mothers when they would interfere with our play time. But there was an unspoken rule that we all had to abide by or face severe consequences: "I can call my mother anything, but you better not say anything bad about her."

When the Therapist Rushes Clinical Progress

Rushing clinical progress can also be reflective of the therapist's unbalanced conflict with expectations. Therapy is not for everyone and yet some therapists are impatient with their couples and cannot tolerate their defenses. Some of these clinicians even exert a great deal of pressure on couples to experience insight or to successfully complete homework assignments or exercises, to no avail. This is caused by the therapist's unbalanced conflict and unrealistically high expectations of the couple. In turn, the couple may feel mistreated or more of a failure than when they first arrived in treatment. If the therapist's conflict with expectations is balanced, the couple will experience a calmer, more confident therapeutic atmosphere, and realistic expectations will prevail.

It would not be unusual for a couples therapist to expect too much from, and quickly become frustrated with, a foreign couple with a significant language barrier. For example, I mistakenly was angry with a young Polish couple who had been in America less than two years. The couple spoke poor English and when I asked them if they had insurance, they said they did not. I then charged the couple my usual fee and the couple scheduled a second appointment. However, just before the second session I received a call from a representative of the insurance company with which I was a long-time provider. To my surprise, the representative preceded to scold me for taking the Polish couple's fee when it was stated very specifically in my contract with the company that I was not to collect any more than the designated co-pay. I was ordered to return the fee that I had collected from the couple under threat of breach of contract.

I tried to explain the situation to the insurance representative, but she wasn't listening. I then became so angry with the couple that I fantasied about refusing to treat them. But I was being unrealistic. Although the representative was too harsh with me, I expected too much of the couple who clearly had no idea whether their insurance covered any therapy. They in fact called the number on the back of their insurance card simply to ask about coverage.

Another example of how cultural difference can impact the expectations of the couples therapist was conveyed to me by a female supervisee who saw herself as a feminist. The supervisee told me that she was treating a mixed-race couple – the husband was from Yemen and the wife was from Sweden – who had recently moved to the United States. According to my supervisee, the couple presented for treatment because the wife felt that her husband was unbearably controlling and treated her as if she was a subservient Middle Eastern woman. No matter how many times she tried to tell her husband that he could not dominate her as he did women in his country of origin, he refused to accept that he was doing anything wrong.

While a case like this is hard enough for the most objective therapist to maintain balance and treat, my supervisee lost perspective and was enraged with the husband's macho attitude towards his wife. In response, and against my advice, she took up the wife's cause and challenged the husband's authority. She told me that she expected him to eventually see her perspective, but he never did. The wife decided to divorce her husband and he in turn blamed the therapist.

My supervisee had the unrealistic expectation that she could turn this man against his cultural background, but she was wrong. She was unable to turn this Middle Eastern man into a feminist. Furthermore, she could not believe that he then had the audacity to then blame her for his divorce. I gently told her that perhaps she expected this man to give up too much of himself. Her out-of-control conflict cost her the treatment.

Change is hard, and some clients are either too fragile or defended to benefit from psychotherapy. Others may be better suited to complete a course of individual therapy and return to couples therapy later, if still needed. But in the name of balance, if one partner is referred for individual treatment the other should be as well (Berman, 1982). The main point, however, is that the therapist who expects couples to progress smoothly through the therapeutic process without setbacks is being quite unrealistic.

The Therapist's Worst Fantasy

Perhaps the most controversial expectation and miscalculation on the therapist's part is that he/she can get romantically or sexually involved with a client and all will end well. This is without a doubt a malfunction in the therapist's conflict with expectations and research findings support this. Pope and Vetter (1991) conducted a large-scale national study and found that 90% of the patients who were sexually involved with a therapist were harmed; 80% were harmed when the sexual involvement began after termination; 11% required hospitalization; 14% attempted suicide; and 1% committed suicide. Therapists who have sex with their clients also run the risk of being reported to their respective licensing boards which may revoke or suspend their license to practice. There is also the risk of legal claims, as well as the loss and respect of their colleagues and family members. This is more likely to happen when a therapist tries to end the relationship.

Surprisingly, when exposed, many therapists (7% of the perpetrators are male compared to 1.5% female) (Pope, 2001) experience shock in part, because they could not imagine that the client would report them to the authorities. A male therapist I had treated – after he was sanctioned – admitted that he specifically told a female client that he would only engage in an affair with her if she promised not to ever tell anybody. When she agreed, he proceeded with the relationship and trusted that it would never be revealed. But as is common, the relationship dissolved by his hand, the client hired an attorney who advised her that she could sue and make a substantial amount of money. When I questioned the therapist about his misplaced trust, he said that he never expected this woman under any circumstances to report him. He said he thought she was too in love with him to do such a thing. His conflict got the best of him.

A particularly egregious act takes place when a couples therapist has sexual relations with one of the partners of a couple. And there are several reasons for this: 1) they are supposed to be helping the couple with their relationship, not trying to wreck it; 2) unlike individual therapy, the couples therapist knows both partners and should have equal allegiances to both; and 3) the couples therapist must regularly face the partner he/she is betraying, rendering the entire treatment process illegitimate. For the couples therapist to expect empathy, especially from the innocent partner, is unrealistic given the pain it causes the couple. The act itself is representative of the therapist's unbalanced conflict because it sabotages the treatment and all those involved.

When the Therapist Expects Too Little from Couples

When the couples therapist expects too little from clients it may show in the structuring of the treatment process and be representative of a dysfunctional conflict. Therapists who expect too little usually underestimate the couple's abilities in any number of contexts. For example, they may underestimate a couple's ability to take responsibility for their treatment. This can manifest in allowing the couple to negotiate lower fees than they can afford, cancel sessions at the last minute, or fail to show without warning. The therapist might also do the bulk of the work in treatment, saving the couple stress but inadvertently blocking their ability to function independently. This is evident when the therapist does most of the talking or allows the couple to continuously ask questions. Tactics such as these may be unconsciously employed by the couple as a defense to keep the therapist from examining them too closely. In this sense the best defense is considered a good offense.

Therapists who expect too little from their clients may also fail to challenge them appropriately. I have been told by more than one supervisee that my style is too confrontive, even harsh at times. But I have found that these same budding clinicians allow clients to sit in their offices for years without any progress. These individuals may value themselves as "nice" caretakers but in my experience a couple will respect them more if they are able to help them overcome their core problems and not babysit them.

When I was a first-year graduate student I was treating a middle-aged man who clearly had anger for women. When the man spoke of them, he would tell me in the crudest way what he would like to do to them sexually. He used his fist in an obscene way to make his point. When I reported this to my supervisor, she asked me how I responded. I told her that I just listened to the man because I wanted to avoid angering him any further. With that, my supervisor – a woman in her 60s – took her glasses off, put them on her desk, and starred at me for a moment. She then leaned over, looked me straight in the eyes and said: "Look you, therapy is a tough business and if you can't confront a misogynist do us all a favor and find some other profession."

Years later a clinical trainee that I was responsible for was told to collect fees from his couples following each session. The clinic relied on this money to pay its staff and to survive. However, the trainee regularly neglected to charge a particular couple because he said he felt sorry for them. When I challenged him on his enabling and lack of objectivity, he became belligerent and accused me of having a "cold heart." The trainee was almost kicked out of the training program for not abiding by the training institute's fee policy. He was also accused of practicing "bad couples therapy" (Doherty, 2002, p. 26) for enabling the couple, and by helping to replicate their chaotic dynamic in the treatment setting; the same dysfunctional dynamic that supports their unbalanced conflict of getting their needs met. While the trainee was pondering whether to maintain his stance or to abide by clinic rules, he discovered that the couple was unwilling to pay even the smallest fee. It was then that he realized that expecting too little of them was problematic. He also realized that he "almost" sacrificed his career in exchange for caretaking a couple that did not seem to care what he had to risk.

The Dynamics of the Therapist's Conflict

If the therapist has a conflict with expectations and it is unbalanced, the therapist, like each partner of the couple, will vacillate between having their expectations met and being disappointed. For example, a therapist may agree to treat a couple that can barely afford the fee and expect them to pay but become disappointed in them when they can't.

Some therapists make the mistake of accepting a couple who live in a geographically undesirable location only to be disappointed with them for missing sessions or failing altogether to continue treatment. While it is flattering to think that you are a good enough therapist to merit a long drive, the odds are low that it will work in the long run.

A woman called from a neighboring state and insisted that I treat her even though I offered her referrals in her city. After two sessions, however, she and her husband dropped out of therapy citing traffic problems. Fortunately, I escaped disappointment because I was skeptical about the possibility of success to begin with.

Sometimes couples fool the therapist into giving them an appointment by insisting that they are invested in making their relationship work. Couples therapists love to hear something like this and get their hopes up that they will have a relatively easy case with a good outcome. But once the couple present for treatment and the therapist sees that there is very little commitment from one or both partners, the therapist may become deflated. The following example better illustrates specifically how a young supervisee made the mistake of not setting limits and enabled a celebrity couple's shared conflict with expectations. The couple's wealth and fame exacerbated her conflict with expectations, rendering her therapeutically impotent:

Jill: How do you want to be paid?

Therapist: You can mail a check when you're ready. There's no rush.

Jill: Okay. But let's get into it. Time is money.

Liam: Right. Jill is no longer affectionate. Sometimes I think she has lost her attraction for me. She never kisses me hello or goodbye or snuggles with me. We have sex once a week, but it feels like she is just doing her duty.

Jill: He's right but there is a reason. He flirts with every girl he sees, and he makes me feel like an old woman.

Liam: It's no big deal. It's just me. I'm not doing anything wrong. Get over it.

Therapist: Liam, you complain that you want Jill to be more affectionate with you but your response to her pain is to "get over it." I can't tell whether you want Jill to meet your expectations or not.

Liam: I think both of you are making too big a deal out of this. I can't help it that I'm famous and women want to flirt with me. Besides, it's good for business.

Therapist: What business is that, show business or the marriage business?

Jill: It's certainly not good for our marriage.

Therapist: Jill, do you think that distancing from Liam is good for the marriage?

Jill: Probably not but I can't give him what I don't feel like giving him.

Therapist: You both express what you think the other should be doing to make things better but neither of you follow through. But you both hold cards that the other wants. How can you both have your expectations met if you refuse to compromise?

Several sessions have gone by without payment. And even though the therapist was becoming increasingly anxious, she was reticent to challenge the couple. Finally, she could not take it anymore and gently addressed the issue.

Therapist: Uh, no pressure, but I haven't received any payments yet. I would hate for you two to fall too far behind.

Liam: [Laughing]. Don't worry, we're good for it. Besides we can handle any bill you throw at us. But I'll get on it.

Jill: Yeah. You know where to find us.

Therapist: Okay. No problem.

As is indicative of a conflict with expectations, the therapist "did" want the couple to pay their balance, but she refrained from pressing the issue and showing its importance in the therapeutic process. For example, she could have tried to link the couple's unpaid balance and their cavalier attitude towards therapist's needs, to their inability to meet each other's needs, but her conflict prevented this. Instead, she enabled the couple by allowing them to ignore her needs, the way they ignore each other. But this is the power of an unbalanced conflict. No matter whether you are a client or a therapist, all people have master conflicts and when balanced they cause little if any problems, and only for a brief time at worst. But if the master conflict is not under control or out-of-balance, it can cause serious problems in a relationship, and in a wide variety of other contexts. You can bet on it.

References

Berman, E. (1982). The individual interview as a treatment technique in conjoint therapy. *American Journal of Family Therapy, 10*, 27–37.

Betchen, S. (205). *Intrusive partners elusive mates: The pursuer-distancer dynamic in couples*. Routledge.

Doherty, W. (2002). Bad couples therapy: How to avoid doing it. *Psychotherapy Networker, 26,* 26–33.

Freud, S. (1937/1964). Analysis Terminable and Interminable. In J. Strachey (Ed. And Trans.), *The standard edition of the complete psychological works of Sigmund Freud* (Vol. 23, pp. 216–253). Hogarth Press and the Institute of Psychoanalysis.

Fromm-Reichmann, F. (1950). *Principles of intensive psychoanalytic psychotherapy*. University of Chicago Press.

Pope, K. (2001). Sex between therapists and clients. In J. Worell (Ed.), *Encyclopedia of women and gender: Sex similarities and differences and the impact of society on gender* (pp. 955–962). Academic Press.

Pope, K., & Vetter, V. (1991). Prior therapist-patient sexual involvement among patients seen by psychologists. *Psychotherapy: Theory, Research, Practice, Training, 28,* 429–438. https://doi.org/10.1037/0033-3204.28.3.429

Weeks, G., & Fife, S. (2014). *Couples in treatment: Techniques and approaches for effective practice* (3rd ed.). Routledge.

Weeks, G., Odell, M., & Methven, S. (2005). *If only I had known...avoiding common mistakes in couples therapy*. Norton.

Epilogue

There were two main points in this book: 1) to explore an important issue facing couples that rarely gets attention in the professional literature and its conflicting complexities: unmet expectations; and 2) to promote the integration of couples and sex therapy in demonstrating how to assess and treat unmet expectations with both nonsexual and sexual symptoms. On the first point, one of the best compliments I ever received from a supervisor was that I did not write for the sake of publishing as much material as I could to pad my resume. She believed that I wrote only when I found a concept interesting enough to merit attention, and when I believed that it would benefit the clinical work of fellow couples therapists. This is true on both counts. In my 40 plus years of treating couples suffering from a wide variety of problems, two concepts have long dominated my thinking, especially in the context of internal conflict: "control struggles" and "unmet expectations." At least one of these concepts always seemed to be a confounding factor in a couple's symptomatology and thus worthy of greater attention. While some therapists may debate the point, I believe it would be hard for any of them to totally discount the importance of control and expectation in relationships.

With respect to integration, it still escapes me why professionals in the field of marriage and family therapy neglect the obvious need to integrate marriage/couples and sex therapy. Perhaps it is because this would require more training, or because some therapists are uncomfortable with the concept of sex. I have had supervisees request couples' supervision but tell me they did not wish to discuss a couple's sexual problems. They would rather refer the case to someone else.

On the other hand, there are those therapists that fancy themselves sex therapists that lack training in couples therapy. This is equally puzzling because sex tends to happen between two individuals. I do realize that there are fewer supervisors with expertise in both disciplines, and the programs that train prospective therapists in both couples and sex therapy are few and far between. But they do exist and, in my opinion, are worth the effort.

A couple's relational problems can reveal a lot about a couple's sex life and *vice versa*. For example, I was giving a talk at a teaching institute on some of the basic sexual disorders. I happened to lead off with a case in which the husband suffered from delayed ejaculation.

After a few descriptive words about the case, a well-respected senior member of the clinic asked from the back of the room if the husband withheld his feelings from his wife. When I inquired as to why she chose to ask that question she answered that men who withhold their feelings are likely to also withhold a part of themselves – in this case their ejaculation. When I told her that the man did in fact have trouble expressing himself, she then asked me if he was frugal as well, and for the same reason. I was fascinated by this exchange and to this day I see the inextricable linkage between sex and relational dynamics. I am completely sold on the integration between these two fields and will continue to pursue it across different relevant concepts such as expectations.

In terms of future clinical study, I do believe that there are other important concepts that should be explored in the context of couples' work. I am especially struck when people form long-term relationships or marry for precarious reasons that will not provide them with genuine security and stability. In some relationships, both partners are conscious of the risk they are taking while in others only one of them might be.

It is especially startling and worth examining when both partners choose to get into a precarious relationship consciously. Perhaps my most stark example of this was that of a man in his 60s who decided to marry a woman in her 30s. This man was a plumber with a high-school education and his new wife held a master's degree in engineering. The man looked every bit his age and his wife presented as energetic, youthful, and vivacious. She even moved twice as fast as he did and showed a curiosity about life that her husband lacked. In the middle of a marital crisis, with his wife threatening to leave him, the man admitted to me in an individual session (his wife was visiting relatives) that he never thought that his marriage would last more than five years. Now that it is approaching its end, he said, he can live with it. He described his situation as being like an old-fashioned egg timer, and his time had run out. He said he had a great time while it lasted, and he held no animosity towards his wife. It was interesting to discover that when she returned to couples therapy, the wife also admitted she knew the marriage would not last prior to marrying.

Other people are conscious that their choice leaves much to be desired but may believe they can tolerate it indefinitely. The following is an example in which only one partner is aware of the precariousness of his relationship. A man who claimed that he could never say "no" to anyone, succumbed to family pressure and married a woman he was not in love with. While he tolerated his situation for a time, however, he soon began an affair with someone he met online. The woman he was having an affair with fit his tastes and he was wildly attracted to her. He eventually left his wife – who claimed to have no clue he felt this way- and remarried his lover. He was conscious of his choice and knew from the start that the relationship but erroneously thought he could live it.

A similar example is that of a woman who only "liked" her husband but married him when she was young and needy. This man had a large family and she felt safe and secure with them. But because the marriage was out of need and not emotional and physical attraction it fell apart as soon as the woman became independent. This woman knew that she was not physically and sexually attracted to her husband, but she was mistaken in thinking she could stay married under these conditions. Her husband was in shock when she told him that she was leaving him.

If at least one partner of a couple was "never" physically attracted to the other, I believe it is near impossible for this attraction to grow, unless the partner was initially repressing the attraction. However, if this partner was once attracted to the other and for some reason lost it (e.g., the other had an affair), I believe this partner can with great effort, find it again (Betchen, 2013, 2015, 2019).

A student argued that she initially saw someone as a friend only to become attracted to them at a later point in time. In cases like these, I believe that the attraction was there to begin with; the student merely repressed her attraction for some reason. If it never existed, it would never have been able to surface.

A man and woman who had been friends for years developed what she referred to as a platonic relationship. Even though he was a handsome young man to whom she had a lot in common she never considered him a romantic partner. At a party one evening a girlfriend of hers commented that this man was sexy. That, according to the woman, opened her eyes, and she began to see this man in a romantic light. Soon the couple started dating. There is, however, data to support my hypothesis. First, the woman had been traumatized by a previous relationship and she was defending against entering another one. Second, even though the two got together, they did not last more than a couple of months. They even broke up and came back together but to no avail, suggesting a lack of a deeper connection that one might find in mutually attracted partners. People that are emotionally and physically attracted to each other have difficulty letting go so easily.

Sometimes only one partner might consciously get into a relationship with no intent of staying. A military man met his wife while stationed in an Eastern Bloc country. She was from a poor family and made it clear that her dream was to one day come to the United States. Finding her intriguing and very attractive the serviceman immediately married this woman and transferred back to the US. But as soon as his new bride learned the language and obtained college and professional degrees, she immediately divorced him. He said he was surprised but she began to avoid him the closer she got to completing her studies. "I knew something was up when she stopped having sex with me," he said. "At first, I thought it was because she was focused on finishing her studies. But I then saw that she was preparing to leave me. I feel like an idiot."

Given these examples, it should not be hard to see the value in exploring the precarious reasons some people give when choosing a long-term partner. When people marry for the wrong reasons, many others beyond the partnership could get hurt such as children and other family members. Still, I notice that most therapists tend to stay away from this subject area, and I suspect it is because of a fear of failure. While therapists are truth seekers, they do hate to fail. Research indicates that therapists experience a sense of demoralization when treatment fails (Swift & Greenberg, 2015). Others feel sadness, confusion, disappointment, and shame (Piselli et al., 2011). Moola (2016) believed that some therapists symbolically take on the role of a parent in the life of the client and react accordingly. If this is true and therapists are ignoring this area, the more reason to study it.

References

Betchen, S. (2013, November). The role of physical attraction in your relationship: Can you get it if you've never had it? Retrieved from www.psychologytoday.com/bloig/magnetic-partners/201311/the-role-physical-attraction-in-your-relationship

Betchen, S. (2015, September). Why we marry people we aren't physically attracted to: The importance of laying a good relational foundation. Retrieved from www.psychologytoday.com/blog/magnetic-partners/201509/why-we-marry-people-we-arent-physically-attracted

Betchen, S. (2019, August). How to tell your partner you are not physically attracted: Are you having trouble revealing this to your partner? Retrieved from www.psychologytoday.com/us/blog/magnetic-partners/201908/how-tell-your-partner-you-are-not-physically-attracted

Moola, F. (2016). Therapeutic endings: Reflections on the treatment of counseling-based research relationships among patients with cystic fibrosis and their caregivers. *Society, Gender Studies & Cultural Studies, 28*, 358–374. https://doi.org/10/1177/0961463X16631765

Piselli, A., Halgin, R. P., & MacEwan, G. H. (2011). What went wrong? Therapists' reflections on their role in premature termination. *Psychotherapy Research, 21*, 400–415. https://doi.org/10.1080/10503307.2011.573819

Swift, J. & Greenberg, R. (2015). Improving psychotherapy effectiveness by addressing the problem of premature termination: Introduction to a special section. *Psychotherapy Research, 28*, 669–671. https://doi.org./10.1080/10503307.2018.1439192

Index